THE ANIMALS IN MY LIFE

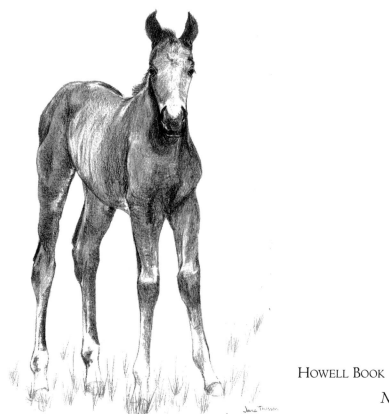

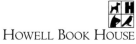

HOWELL BOOK HOUSE

New York

THE ANIMALS
IN MY LIFE

Stories of a Country Vet

GRANT KENDALL
Drawings by Jane Thissen

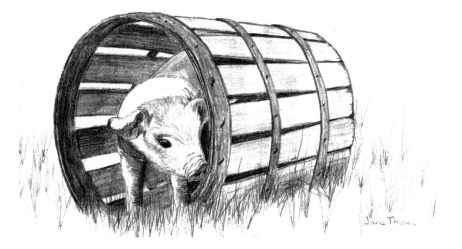

All the stories in this book are true, however, the names of the people and animals have been changed.

Howell Book House
A Simon & Schuster Macmillan Company
1633 Broadway
New York, NY 10019

MACMILLAN is a registered trademark of Macmillan, Inc.

Library of Congress Cataloging-in-Publication Data
Kendall, Grant.
        The animals in my life : stories of a country vet / Grant Kendall.
        p. cm.
ISBN: 0-87605-746-6
1. Kendall, Grant. 2. Veterinarians—United States—Biography. 3. Animals—United States—Anecdotes. I. Title.
SF613.K45 1996
636.089'092—dc20
[B]   95-50587
        CIP

Manufactured in the United States of America
10 9 8 7 6 5 4 3

For Kristin and Jennifer

CONTENTS

INTRODUCTION

Being a veterinarian is fun and sure beats working for a living. Most of the time, though, the work is routine, even mundane, and requires only the same tasks repeated over and over, day after day. For instance, I may do nothing at all for days except examine mares.

This is hardly an exciting, amusing or even eventful pastime (unless the mare should kick, at which point it still isn't amusing), and stories written about this would be pretty boring and lack any entertainment value. Fortunately, other things happen from time to time that are worth sharing, and they interrupt the daily routine often enough to make veterinary medicine a great life.

Unfortunately, in relating these incidents to non-vet-oriented readers, words such as *palpate, ovulate* and *farrow* pop up and may not be understood by everyone. There are other words, such as *twitch* and *jump*, which are in everyday usage but which mean something entirely different when applied to vet work. They are all necessary to relate the stories, but rather than force the reader to refer to a dictionary or, worse, read lengthy explanations in the middle of a story, I have provided a glossary.

Being a vet does not limit one only to animal contact. Each animal has an owner or at least someone responsible for it, and these people are as big a part of veterinary practice as their animals are. Every animal has its own personality, just as every person does, but just as every person's story would not make for interesting reading, most animals' stories would bore you to tears. Some stand out, though—both animals and people—and their stories follow.

Part One

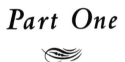

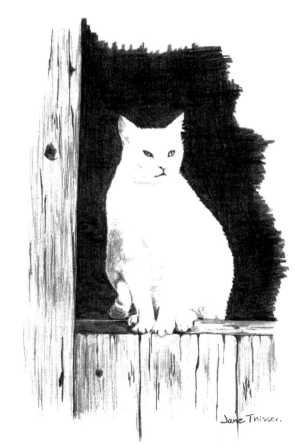

Jane Thissen.

FLIPPER

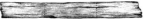

There was a purpose for Flipper, but it took a long time to find it.

I was in my senior year in vet school, and money was a problem. My wife taught school, and I worked two jobs at the college. My first job was for one of the professors, Dr. Barker, caring for a kennel of dogs in which he was studying inherited diseases. I also helped a little in his research. The job required about two hours each weekday and maybe another two or three hours on weekends.

The other job was also about twelve or fifteen hours a week, but only on weekends. I worked for the Laboratory Animal Department, and my job was cleaning cages and feeding the research animals: rats, mice, guinea pigs, etc. Part of this department was the local dog pound, where strays were brought and kept for a couple of weeks to see if they would be claimed or adopted. It was my job to clean and feed this area on weekends.

This was not a pleasant part of the job. I knew what would happen to these dogs after two weeks if no one wanted them, and though I tried not to think about it, sometimes I did in spite of myself.

Each Saturday morning when I showed up to clean the runs, there would be a few new dogs, and a few that I remembered from the previous Sunday would be gone. I tried to tell myself that those that were missing had found good homes, but I knew better. The trip to Lab Animal was almost always a one-way journey.

One Saturday morning when I stepped into one of the runs, a little, short-haired brown and white dog ran up to me. This in itself was unusual; most of the animals were frightened in their strange surroundings and stayed far away from me.

But this little dog, maybe twenty pounds, acted as if I was her best friend, and she leaped on me and yapped and wanted as much attention as she could get me to give her.

And she was obviously very pregnant.

I petted her awhile and then went on about my work. As I went from run to run, she kept watching me and calling to me. I finished the twenty or so runs, then went back to hers and petted her a little more.

The next morning when I returned, she once again greeted me as if I was all she'd ever wanted. Her desire for affection was tremendous. A few hours later, when my work was done, I went back to see her. And again she was ecstatic.

During the week I thought about her. I had no way of knowing when she would have her puppies, but it couldn't be much longer. In the middle of the week I looked in on her, and again she welcomed me with all her enthusiasm. By now she was developing milk, and her little udders were almost full.

The next Saturday the story was the same. I didn't know what day she had arrived, but because she had been there the previous Saturday, I knew she would *not* be there the next Saturday.

Because of our situation at home—we already had two dogs— we really could not afford another one at that time, but something had to be done for this little gal. I thought about it all that day and made my decision.

The next morning—Sunday—I removed her from the run. Maybe she wouldn't be missed; after all, each run contained from four to eight dogs. I took her to Dr. Barker's research kennel and placed her in an empty run there.

On Monday morning I approached Dr. Barker. "Doc," I said, "I've picked up a little stray and put her in your kennel. Is that okay?"

"Why don't you take her to Lab Animal? That's where the strays go," he replied.

"Well, that's where I picked her up," I confessed, and explained the situation. He understood, but cautioned me. "You know you can probably get in trouble for this if someone hears about it, maybe lose your Lab Animal job."

I assured him that I was aware of the potential consequences.

"Okay," he said, "but try to do something with her soon. She'll be hard to explain if she's found there."

That was of little concern—he and I were the only ones who went to his kennel—but I told him I would find a home for her as soon as I could.

However, she beat me to the punch. The next day she whelped three pups: one mostly white female, one mostly brown female, and one brown and white male, marked almost exactly like her.

The two little girls were bright, healthy, normal puppies, but the male, although bright and apparently healthy, was *not* normal. He had no front legs, just very small stumps at the shoulders.

I showed the pups to Dr. Barker. "You better put that one to sleep," he said, pointing to the male. "He'll never make it like that."

I agreed that his future looked bleak, but somehow I couldn't see saving his mother just to kill him when he was born. I said so to Dr. Barker.

"Suit yourself. It'll just be more difficult when he's older." Again he stressed the importance of finding a home for this family.

I named the pups, showing great originality. I called the white one Whitey and the brown one Brownie. The boy I called Flipper.

Flipper handled himself very well with his sisters. He was able to get to his mom to nurse and generally acted like any other puppy.

Dr. Barker had warned me to be on the alert for other problems with Flipper; often, he told me, if there was one birth defect there might be another one, one that might not be so apparent.

A couple of weeks passed, and it was time for their eyes to open. Brownie's opened first, then the next day Whitey opened hers. But Flipper's didn't open, not even a little bit. Oh boy, I thought, was this going to be the other problem? Would he be blind?

Two more days passed, and still nothing. I was afraid to tell Dr. Barker; I knew what he would say. But on the third day, Flipper's left eye glistened a little between the lids. Then the next day the right one also sneaked a peek at the world. Two more days and they were both fully open.

But now Whitey and Brownie were walking. At least, they were standing and wobbling. Flipper still crawled around like a snake, occasionally pushing himself a little with his hind legs.

He began having a hard time nursing. His sisters could use their little front legs as pushers, clearing a path to the dinner table, but Flipper couldn't push back and was usually jostled aside as the girls nursed their fill. But his mother was very patient. After the other two were satisfied and fell off to sleep, Mama would just lie there, and that's when Flipper could nurse in peace.

As more time passed, Brownie and Whitey were getting around well, bouncing and running and wrestling, but Flipper still just slithered. One day Dr. Barker called me into his office. "I was just out to the kennel. That puppy is not going to be able to have a decent life. When are you going to do something about it?"

I assured him that something would be done soon, but when I said it I thought I was lying.

Two days later, something *was* done. I went out to feed the dogs and was greeted pretty much as usual. Mama ran out, as delighted as ever to see somebody, followed by the bounding pair of females. But right behind them came Flipper.

He was hopping like a kangaroo!

Somehow he had balanced himself on his hind legs, from the feet to the hocks, and was using his tail as a sort of rudder. He bounced up right behind the others. Stopping was a problem; he fell on his nose when he applied the brakes but hopped right up again on his hocks.

As the days went by he became more proficient at this mode of locomotion, using his tail less and less for balance.

I was earnestly trying to find homes for all four of them now. Dr. Barker said they had to go, so I was taking my classmates, veterinary students all, to see them, hoping someone would want one or all. And it worked, almost. Brownie was the first to go, to one of my friends as a gift for his wife. Then Whitey was taken by a student in the class behind mine, who took her to his parents' home for his little brother. Even the little mother dog, whom I had only called Mama, found a home with one of my female classmates.

But no one would take Flipper. Each person I brought to see him would be hailed with such affection and adoration that I thought it would be impossible for him to be turned down. Everyone thought he was wonderful and loved his personality, but no one would give him a home.

Flipper was now alone in the large dog run. I worried about that, so I approached Dr. Walken, who was in charge of the school's Small Animal Clinic. I told him about Flipper and asked if I could move him into one of the large cages in the clinic. He would have more company, and more importantly, I thought, be seen by more people, thus increasing his chances of adoption.

Dr. Walken went with me to see him. He was amazed at this little seven-week-old puppy's ability, coordination and, most of all, friendliness. He assigned a cage to me to keep him in, but cautioned that his care was mine; it would not be the responsibility of the students working in the clinic.

It was not long before Flipper was the center of attention of the entire vet school. Over two hundred students and faculty members came to care for him, and he loved them all. But, still, no one would take him home. They'd take him out and play with him, but, always, they put him back in his cage and left him.

I always brought my lunch, and on nice days I'd sit out on the grass to eat. And I'd take Flipper out with me. He would hop around like a rabbit among the bushes and joyfully greet anyone who happened by.

One day while we were outside, one of my classmates walked up. Jamie Bell was his name, and even though we had been together in school for more than three years, I really didn't know him. No one did. Jamie was a loner, a very quiet loner, so I was quite surprised when he spoke to me.

"Hi, Grant."

"Hi, Jamie," I replied. "How's everything?"

He ignored my attempt at small talk. "Does Flipper have a home yet?" he asked.

Flipper was almost four months old now, and still there had been no takers. "No, Jamie, and it's not looking good. I think his welcome is wearing thin, too. The clinic is crowded, and they'll need his cage soon."

"I might know someplace that will want him. I'm going home this weekend. I'll ask." And he turned and walked off.

I called to him, asking him to tell me more, but he just kept on walking.

The weekend passed, and on Monday I looked for Jamie. "Did you ask about Flipper?" I asked when I finally found him.

"Yes. They'd like to see him. Can we take him there next weekend?"

"Where?"

"To the place that may want him."

"Yes, but where? And can't they come here?"

"It's a lot of people, and it's a ways off."

It had never occurred to me before, but I didn't know where Jamie was from. After three-plus years of constant exposure, we learn a lot about our classmates. I at least knew the state, if not the city, most of them called home, but I had no idea where Jamie lived.

"Where is this place, Jamie?" I asked.

"Right near home," and he named a city nearly three hundred miles away. At least six hours each way! "We can leave after classes Friday," he continued. "We'll be there by ten or eleven. We can come back Saturday afternoon, if you want. I think they'll like him."

"Who are these people? I'd like to know before I blow a weekend."

"They're just some people who might want Flipper. Really."

I'm not sure why, but I agreed to go with him. We arranged everything for Friday, and I set about finding someone to work for me that weekend, the whole weekend just in case we didn't get back Saturday night.

On Friday afternoon around four-thirty, we threw our stuff in my car, an Opel station wagon (much roomier than Jamie's VW Beetle), putting Flipper in a pet carrier in the back seat; it was his first time in a car and I feared car sickness. After about fifty miles it looked pretty certain that he wouldn't get sick, so I told Jamie to let him out.

He hopped into the front seat with us, renewed acquaintances and then went to sleep in Jamie's lap.

It was an uneventful trip. Flipper slept most of the way, and Jamie didn't say ten words. I kept questioning him about these people who were interested in Flipper, but he said it would be better if I waited to see them.

We pulled into Jamie's parents' driveway at about ten forty-five, and Flipper and I were shown to the spare room, where an unbelievably miserable hide-a-bed awaited me. Flipper spent the night in his pet carrier and I think he rested well. I didn't.

Early the next morning—Saturday—we headed out to see the people who might want Flipper. We drove more than twenty miles, Jamie directing me; finally he told me to turn into the next drive. It led back to a very large, very old house. Next to the house was a parking lot with spaces for maybe twenty cars, and all around the property was a high chain-link fence. This was not an ordinary residence.

We put Flipper back in his carrier and carried him to the front door. On the grass just before we stepped onto the porch was a small sign: "Home for Handicapped Children."

Jamie rang the bell, and a pleasant-looking, chubby woman of maybe thirty-five came to the door.

"Hi, Mrs. Watson," Jamie greeted her. "This is my friend Grant, and this"—he pointed to the carrier—"is the puppy I told you about."

We were greeted warmly and invited in.

"The children are all in the back room," she told us. "Just bring him back and we'll see what happens."

We walked down a short hallway, through a large double door and into a big room in which twelve to fourteen children were sitting. Some were young, maybe three or four, and the oldest appeared to be in her mid-teens.

And they were, indeed, handicapped. It was a depressing sight, all of these kids sitting there quietly, looking very apprehensive.

"Children," Mrs. Watson began, "Jamie and his friend have brought someone for you to meet."

I opened the carrier and Flipper hopped out. He sped to the nearest child, a girl of about ten in a wheelchair, and bounced into her lap, where he immediately began to lick her face from top to bottom. At first the child screeched, then she realized it wasn't an attack and began to laugh.

Then Flipper leaped down and went off to see who else he had to meet. One by one he visited each child, bounding around the room. A very small boy cried at first, but when he saw that everyone else was delighted, he, too, joined in the laughter.

We stayed for about two hours, and Flipper loved the attention.

When it was time to go, Mrs. Watson took us aside and told us it seemed he would almost certainly work out fine, but, "Can we try it tonight and see what happens by tomorrow?"

We left Flipper's food and bowls, gave her general puppy-care instructions and told her we'd be back early Sunday morning. As we left, I told Jamie I was impressed with his choice. As usual, he just sat there.

The next morning, after another night on the hide-a-bed from Hades, we went back to the Home. As we entered the hallway leading to the big room, we heard shouting and laughter and Flipper's name being called.

We went into the room and he saw us. He bounced over on his little hind legs and leaped up and down until I picked him up. He wiggled and licked and then jumped down and hopped back to the children.

"The only problem we had," Mrs. Watson said, "was the argument over whom he would sleep with. We'll have to make a schedule."

We only stayed a short time, and as I turned to leave, I felt tears coming. I said, "Bye, Flipper," and he came over to me for just a second, then returned to his children. I knew there was no better place for him.

As we left, I asked Mrs. Watson to keep me posted on him. I received a letter a year from her. She told me that Flipper would greet new children who came to the Home just as he had greeted the kids on that first day, and that even as an adult and then as an old dog, he retained his zest for life and his love for people.

The children who came to the Home were usually insecure and frightened, not understanding what was happening to them. Flipper was their therapy, helping to make the difficult adjustment much easier for them. This was evidently Flipper's purpose for being here—to show these children how to get by in the world with their own disabilities.

The saddest news I've ever received in my life was a short note from Mrs. Watson several years ago. Flipper, fifteen years old, had died in his sleep.

COWS

I don't care for cows. By that, I mean not only do I not tend to their health problems, I also don't particularly like them.

I didn't always dislike them, however. For the first twenty-five years or so of my life I had no feelings about them at all. My entire knowledge of the species was gleaned from Saturday double-feature matinees, one of the great pleasures of youth denied to the children of today.

One of these movies each Saturday involved the "driving"— a misleading term because no cars were connected with this undertaking—of a herd of cattle from someplace in Texas to the railhead in Dodge City, which was usually in Kansas.

I never understood why this was being done. It certainly couldn't have been for the benefit of the cattle or the cowboys, unless you can call beneficial the stampede, created by thunder and lightning, that would occur on the third or fourth day out at a point too far from home for the cowboys to say "the heck with it," so they went out and chased the cows down rather than pack up and leave.

I guess this long trip *was* beneficial to the rustlers, though. How would they have made a living if the cows simply had caught a train down in Texas or if they had actually been raised in the Kansas countryside around Dodge City? I mean, if the cows only had to walk two miles to catch their train, what chance would an honest rustler have?

And that was it. That was my total knowledge of cows. I knew milk came from them, sure, but the milk arrived in glass or cardboard containers, and the only hint of cow contact was the stenciled head of one on the side of a carton.

So I was well advanced in college before I ever had person-to-cow contact. This momentous event occurred when I was taking a course called Beef Production. Herein we learned that cows are an early form of pot roast, and occasionally we were taken out to the university farm to actually look upon this pre-beef.

Later we were introduced to a little cow care. Basically, we were shown how to get a cow into a chute, at the end of which was a headgate. This is a device the cow put her head through just as someone pushed a lever, which would close the contraption around her neck, thereby trapping her and enabling the person in question to do various things to her.

This was tricky in itself. The cows did not like to have their heads trapped—can you blame them?—and would either not proceed down the chute at all or would proceed at such a rapid pace that only the quickest, most coordinated lever-manipulator could react in time to catch them.

The cows probably enjoyed this exercise with our class more than they did with most, since we were a singularly inept group. More often than not we were unable to react in a timely fashion, and Bossy just leaped on through and hightailed it across the open field.

But we *would* catch the occasional slow or senile animal, and when we did, we were shown how to use nose tongs, a device somewhat reminiscent of a pair of pliers.

Nose tongs were used to hold a cow's head still in case we wanted her to have a still head for some reason, but—and this should not come as a big surprise—the average cow was not fond of having them applied. She would fling her head about wildly, providing us and our tongs with a moving target we were still expected to grasp.

This is where I began to form an opinion on cows. Dr. Strang, our instructor, handed me the tongs. "Here, Kendall, get her," he ordered.

I tried. I'd lunge for her nose and she'd fling her head and I'd miss. After several unsuccessful attempts, I moved in a little closer— too close, however, as she swung her head violently and brought it in contact with mine.

The cow only weighed about eight hundred pounds, but I feel pretty certain that at least five hundred pounds of it was head. In addition to causing severe pain—my pain, I don't know how *she* felt—she broke my glasses.

Perhaps if this cow had just stood there and allowed me to tong her nose I'd have developed a different feeling toward her kind, but right then and there I decided I was not crazy about them.

Still, "dislike" was probably not the word to best describe my feelings. Maybe something milder, like "distaste," better defined my emotions at this point.

I received my degree in Animal Science, and for several years I had no contact at all with cows, not until my junior year in vet school, when we were expected to apply what we had learned the first two years to real live animals. In this third year of learning, we spent actual time with real dogs, real cats, real horses, real pigs and, alas, real cows.

That "alas" was not how I felt then, though. I recalled my previous cow contact, and I do mean "contact," but it had been three years earlier and the pain had subsided since then. Also dimmed by the passage of time was the fact that I had had to take an exam later that day without my glasses, so although I wasn't eager to work on cows, I looked forward to it as a learning experience.

Junior year of vet school was pretty much spent on clinic duty. We'd spend time in the Small Animal clinic working with and on dogs and cats, time in the Food Animal clinic working with and on cows and pigs, time in the Equine clinic working with and on horses, time in the Radiology clinic X-raying anything that needed to be X-rayed and time in the Ambulatory clinic.

This last part should, theoretically, have been the most enjoyable. Three students accompanied a faculty member on trips to area farms to tend to large animals that weren't sick enough or injured enough to be hauled in to the school for hospitalization.

There were three Ambulatory clinicians, Doctors Wilson, Blackthorn and Emmons. Dr. Wilson took the horse calls, Dr. Blackthorn took the cattle calls and Dr. Emmons took whatever the other two didn't. The students rotated among the three—a week with each—so we'd see a cross section of the real world.

Ambulatory happened to be my first clinic, and my first clinician was Dr. Blackthorn. Along with me were fellow students Larry Mallory and Bill Remmenstadt. We reported to Dr. Blackthorn's office at eight A.M. the first day of classes.

Dr. Blackthorn was a laid-back old country boy who took life pretty easily. He greeted us with his typical big smile and twinkling eyes.

"Hey, boys! We only got a couple things on the schedule today. Put on your overalls and we'll get 'em done, and then we can sit around and play some cards."

We headed out in the big four-door pickup truck with the mobile clinic in its bed.

"First place we're goin' is a little farm just outside town," Dr. Blackthorn told us. "We just got a cow to clean there."

"Cleaning" a cow is a euphemism for removing the placenta after she calves. Normally, of course, the placenta removes itself at the time of calving or shortly thereafter, but occasionally the placenta, for one reason or another, remains attached or partly attached to the cow's uterus.

There is a very short and simple description in the textbooks that tells us how to do this. The procedure in real life is neither short nor particularly simple, but at this point I didn't know that.

We arrived at a pretty seedy-looking little old farm. A pretty seedy-looking little old farmer met us at the end of the driveway.

"Howdy, Doc. I see you got a new bunch of kiddies to learn sumpin' to."

"Yeah, sure do, Homer. They get sorrier every time." He grinned at us. "Where's the patient?"

"Got her here in the shed." He pointed to a ramshackle building behind him. "You can get right at her."

"When did she calve, Homer?"

"Oh, I don't know. Three to four days ago, I guess. I figgered she'd drop that thing out anytime, but it just ain't comin'."

I looked at Bill, and he returned my glance. Three or four days! The textbook said to clean the cow if she still retained her placenta the morning after calving.

We walked around to the other side of the shed. It was enclosed by walls on three sides and by several gates on the open side. These gates were tied to support posts with baling twine. I had expected to see a chute and headgate like they had at the university farm, but none were to be seen.

Inside this shed, roughly twelve feet deep by thirty feet long, was a cow. And not a very happy cow. She was tearing around, bellowing and flapping placenta behind her.

"Where's her calf, Homer?" Dr. B asked.

"Oh, he's out in the field. We didn't need him up here for nothin'."

It appeared the cow felt differently but Dr. B just shrugged.

He addressed us. "Boys, we got to get a rope around her neck and snub her to one of these posts here." He motioned to the support poles on the front of the shed.

He went back to the truck and pulled out a long rope with a noose in one end.

"All right now, listen up," he continued. "Kendall, you put this noose around her neck, and Mallory, you pull her snug to a post."

Once again the directions sounded easy, but to do my end of the job it looked as if I would have to get in there with El Toro, while Larry's portion could best be accomplished by standing outside the shed.

"I don't know anything about cows," I protested.

"All you got to know is which end eats and put that loop over it. Now hop in there and do it."

Very carefully I climbed over one of the gates. Bossy was so intent on running in circles she didn't notice me as I crept slowly in her general direction.

She zoomed by and I flung the noose. Lucky things happen; it went right over her head and settled down around her shoulders. And she hadn't even seemed to notice!

"Okay, Mallory," said Dr. B. "Wrap around that post and tighten her down."

About this time the cow realized her space had been infringed upon. She turned and looked at me, then lowered her head and pawed the ground, snorting. It was like an old bullfight movie, except I had no cape and the pretty señorita with the rose in her teeth was somewhere else.

"Pull the rope, Larry," I pleaded. And he did. Slowly. Slooooowly.

I was at one end of the shed and she was at the other. Larry was still calmly wrapping the rope when she charged.

"Pull the rope!" Dr. B and I shouted in unison.

So, moving a little more quickly but still without great speed, he finally got it snubbed tight, but by then Crazy Cow had reached full speed. And she was in about the center of the shed when she ran out of rope.

When she reached the end of the rope, she was flying! The rope was under her, between her legs, and when she hit the limit she flipped, her rear pitching over her head, which could go no further.

With this sudden flinging of her rear end, the placenta came loose from its uterine attachments. It flew through the air directly at me, striking me in the face and chest and knocking me flat on my back.

Remember, this placenta had been hanging there for days. Decomposition had set in, and it was rotting. And stinking!

And old Homer had evidently not been the most meticulous shed cleaner. The floor had probably been mucked out sometime around the close of World War I and was now roughly a foot deep in various ages of cow excrement. This was where I landed.

I was covered on the front with decomposed placenta and on the back with carefully aged manure. Dr. B looked me over. "Kendall, you're a mess," he said. "I'm not sure we can let you in the truck."

He wrote up a bill for old Homer, who pulled out his wallet and paid him. Homer wasn't real happy. "If I'da knowed it woulda come out that easy I wun'ta called," he mumbled.

It was on the drive back to school, during which I sat on a feed sack obtained from Homer, that I made up my mind about cows: I didn't like them. They are abusive, I concluded. And nothing has happened to change that opinion.

There is one further incident that indelibly cemented the following credo in my mind: The Only Good Cow Is a Medium-Rare Cow.

To wit:

I finally got out of vet school and gained honest employment. I was hired by a large-animal practice in northern Virginia and got to work on a lot of horses, which was my goal. Unfortunately, I also got to work on a lot of cows.

There were a lot of dairies in the area, and I had the chance to clean a lot of cows. I actually became more proficient at it than I ever dreamed was possible. And there was ample opportunity to see other cattle problems.

One day I was called to a Holstein dairy run by an aged gentleman who really liked his cows. There were a hundred of them, and they all had names. Most operations gave their cows numbers, which they wore on tags around their necks or in their ears, but these cows wore no identification at all.

Mr. Amos was the old guy's name, and he could tell all his cows apart. There were Flo and Eleanor and Susie and Bess and Sally Ann and on and on. One hundred cows, one hundred names.

Before we proceed any further, let's go over a few differences between horses, noble and beautiful beasts, and cows, vicious and unpredictable fiends.

Horses don't always approve of what we try to do to them, but they are considerate enough to *warn* us before they show their disapproval. If we pay attention, we won't be hurt by a horse. It may be an ear held back, a twitch of the tail, a shift of weight—but it will be something. A horse *will* warn us.

But a cow! A cow will stand there chewing its cud; batting its big, brown, soulful eyes; mooing its soothing lullaby; not flicking an ear or blinking an eye, and then—WHAM!—it has broken your body into a thousand pieces.

And a horse has a nice, long, muscular neck in which to accept intramuscular injections, while a cow has a little bitty short stub of a neck with barely enough muscles to hold its head up. An IM injection in a cow has to be given in the rump.

Now back to Mr. Amos's dairy. On this particular day, not long after graduation, I was there to treat a cow roughly the size of the Astrodome. Her name was Susie, and while I don't now recall the nature of her ailment, it was one that required an IM injection.

I filled my syringe with medication and edged up to Susie's side. "Mr. Amos," I said, "please tail her up."

He did as I requested, and I plunged the needle into her hip. The next thing I knew, I was sprawled on the other side of the barn, and my right leg was flaming in pain! It could not hurt that much and still be attached to my body!

Mr. Amos looked down at me. "I knew she'd do that," he soberly proclaimed. "Tailin' never did work on Susie."

Fighting back the tears, I managed to snap out between moans, "Why didn't you tell me that?!"

"I figgered you knew what you was doin'," he said.

My leg *was* still attached—it wasn't even broken—but that's not the point. The point is this: Susie gave *no* warning—no blink, no ear flick, no weight shift, no nothing. She just kicked. No self-respecting horse would ever do that.

There were other cow attacks on and off over the year and a half I was employed in that practice, but none since I left there. My wife frequently suggests that we buy a couple of calves and raise them.

I'd rather raise alligators.

CYRIL

Pigs are cool. They aren't like cows, which are the most uncool creatures in the universe. I like pigs.

My knowledge of them in my formative years was even more scant than my knowledge of cows. The reader will recall that my cow knowledge was gained at the Saturday matinees. Well, there just were no great pig drives across the prairie to the railhead or sausage factory or wherever pigs of the Old West went, so I went for years knowing *nothing* about the species at all.

My first pig awareness came when someone told me a race horse I had bet on was named after a breed of pig. The horse's name was Poland China; I had thought he was named after Eastern European plates. That was interesting, but real pigs remained alien to me.

Then there was Arnold Ziffel. Arnold, for those of you too young to have seen the great TV show *Green Acres*, was a pig owned (actually adopted) by Fred and Dora Ziffel, who were not pigs. Arnold was wonderful and probably made pig lovers out of a whole generation of sitcom viewers.

Perhaps if the Ziffels had adopted a cow I would feel differently about them today (although I doubt it), but they didn't. Anyone who didn't like Arnold was not to be trusted.

Still, significant (i.e., the real thing) pig contact had not been made. This didn't come until college—actually, my senior year of college.

I had long before decided I was going to be a veterinarian, but vet school was hard to get into, so just in case something happened and I didn't get in or was unable to complete the four-year course, I chose to get a regular undergraduate degree. The degree program I decided to pursue was Animal Science, which basically teaches a student how to farm.

It was during this course of study that many of my animal likes and dislikes were embedded. I developed that early dislike for cows and a definite partiality toward pigs.

The basis for the development of pig-liking was a young lady named Gina. Gina was a Hampshire sow, and she was assigned to me in a required course called Swine Production. As my "assignment," I was required to look in on her at least once a day in the farrowing barn.

This was pretty easy. If she was actually in the act of giving birth, I was to call the herdsman. The chances of a sow being cooperative enough to actually farrow in the few-minutes time frame that her student was present were pretty low, which is why the job of checking was so simple.

Most of my classmates would walk into the farrowing barn during lunch or between classes, look at their sows long enough to see that nothing was going on (approximately five seconds), and then leave. But my classmates didn't have Gina as their sow.

Gina *liked* people. Anytime someone appeared near her pen, she would come over and snort and squeal until she either got the person's attention or the person left. She loved to have her ears scratched and to be rubbed on the forehead.

I would usually check in with her after my last class of the day—midafternoon—and stay for ten or fifteen minutes, most of which were spent scratching or rubbing her. We both enjoyed this.

All pigs, however, are not like Gina. I learned this one afternoon when I went in to check on her.

I visited with her and petted her for a few minutes, then started to leave. As I walked down the row of pig pens I noticed one sow lying down and obviously straining. The sign on the end of her pen read:

SARAH
STUDENT: WESTMORELAND

It was pretty evident, I thought, that she was attempting to deliver a piglet. I had never seen a sow give birth, but I was pretty sure this was how it would look. Bob Westmoreland was one of my classmates and it was his sow, but I had no idea where to find him. I went to the herdsman's office and he wasn't in, so I went back to watch Sarah some more. After another ten minutes she still hadn't produced a piglet. I became a little concerned.

I knew nothing of pig delivery and the herdsman was still absent, so I used the phone in his office to call Dr. Robinson, my adviser, who was also the head of the Animal Science department. I explained what was going on and he told me to call the vet school and ask for a clinician.

I did, and about ten minutes later Dr. John Emery showed up at the farrowing barn. Yes, he said, she was trying to give birth and something must be wrong. He stepped into her pen and walked toward her rear, but she hopped up and faced him. He tried to circle around her, but Sarah wouldn't let him. She pivoted and continued to face him.

"Kendall," he directed, "hop in here and attract her attention and let me see if I can get behind her."

Sarah thought little of these new, two-to-one odds. When she finally felt threatened enough, she decided to even up her chances by eliminating one of her adversaries.

She charged me!

"Run!" shouted Dr. Emery, but the advice wasn't needed. I had already jumped for the edge of the pen, but she caught my right pants leg, tearing off a pretty good hunk. Then she turned on Dr. Emery. He was already over the railing.

"Go to the herdsman's office and see if he has a snare in there," he told me. A hog snare is a wire loop that is placed over the pig's snout and then tightened; it's sort of like a twitch for a horse.

I came back with a snare and Sarah was down and straining again. Dr. Emery tried to catch her snout, but she jumped up immediately when the loop touched her. He tried for several minutes to snare her with no success. Every time he stopped for even a few seconds, she'd lie down and strain.

Finally, the herdsman returned. Dr. Emery told him what was going on.

"Oh, Sarah is just a miserable creature," he said. "She's a good mother, but just awful to work around."

But this fellow knew a lot about pigs and how to handle them. He opened Sarah's gate and ran her down a chute to a pen that put her in very narrow quarters, unable to turn around.

From this point it was quick work. Dr. Emery determined the problem: piglet number one was trying to enter the world sideways, which just wouldn't work. He straightened it out, and within the next half hour eleven new little squealers were in the world.

The next morning, Bob Westmoreland walked up to me just before our Forage Crops class began. He had been out to the farrowing barn and the herdsman had told him of our experiences the day before. Bob chewed me up one side and down the other for "interfering" with his sow. After a five-minute berating, I concluded that Bob and Sarah were made for each other; they were both miserable creatures.

Gina farrowed several days later, but I missed it. She also had eleven, a pretty good-sized litter for the first one. Her personality didn't change, though; she still liked to be scratched and rubbed.

When Swine Production was over, so was my contact with pigs—for a while, anyway.

I entered vet school the next year and learned a bunch of basics, a lot of which I couldn't understand our having to learn.

"Oh, you'll understand in time. You'll see why we teach you all of this," I was told by several faculty members. It's been more than twenty-five years now and I still don't understand why we learned most of it.

But eventually, thank goodness, we were taught the things we were there to learn: medicine and surgery of domestic animals.

Very little was devoted to pigs, though. We did have a course one quarter called Swine Medicine, which taught us about diseases and treatments, but we saw very little in the way of real pigs. We did take one trip out to the area's only "complete" swine operation—all the way from birth to bacon—which was very impressive. The idea of being a pig farmer was not unappealing.

Still, we had minimal actual pig contact. The pig caseload in the Large Animal clinic was very low, and only occasionally was there a pig call on Ambulatory. My group never had one.

The next significant pig contact for me occurred in our own front yard. My wife and I had bought a small home in a little subdivision on the outskirts of town. Beyond our subdivision was only open land and small farms for miles.

At that time, we owned two dogs—Vichy, a Saint Bernard, and Orf, a mutt. In the winter they slept in the house, but in the summer they just stayed out in the fenced backyard.

One warm summer night about three A.M., Orf and Vichy began a racket such as they'd never done before. They were barking and howling and jumping against the chain-link fence.

My wife thought it must be someone trying to break in, but I was pretty sure it was just a possum or raccoon raiding the trash cans, which sat out at the end of the house by the garage.

Dressed in my bathrobe and armed with a flashlight, I ventured forth to scare away the intruder. As I stepped out the front door, I heard a trash can fall over. Now I *knew* it was some sort of wild critter after a free meal.

I walked down the front steps yelling threats to whatever was there: "Get out of here, you rotten little vermin! Get back to the woods where you belong or I'll make a Davy Crockett hat out of you!" Any self-respecting raccoon would, of course, hightail it upon hearing a threat like that.

But the trash can clattering and dog barking continued unabated.

"All right, I warned you!" I hollered, turning the corner of the house to where the trash cans were.

And there stood the biggest pig in the world, calmly dining on whatever we had thrown out earlier, completely unaffected by my threats.

He looked at me as I shone the light in his face. "Snort!" he said, and then went back to his meal.

Now when I say this pig was big, I mean *BIG!* He was every bit of four feet tall, and had to be eight feet long!

Weighing the situation carefully (and quickly) in my mind, I retreated. Rapidly. Gina had been sweet and affectionate, I recalled, but what if this guy was a Sarah type? Discretion being the better part of valor, I withdrew to the safety of the house.

I called the dogs in the back door to try to get them to be quiet—lights were coming on in neighbors' houses—but they were wound up and wouldn't stop.

My wife asked, "What's going on out there?"

"The King Kong of the pig world is eating our trash," I told her, and described the behemoth to her.

"Call the animal shelter and have them come get it," she suggested.

We did, although I was pretty sure they would have neither the vehicle nor the personnel sufficient to handle the situation. We never learned whether they did or not; at three in the morning all we got was a recording telling us to call after eight A.M.

"Call the police," my wife directed. "They'll know what to do."

I did. The voice on the other end of the line didn't sound at all interested in or alarmed by our situation.

"Pig in garbage," it yawned. "Okay, we'll send a car."

This was about three-twenty. The dogs were still going crazy, and Orf was trying to get out the front door. I'm not sure how good a match this would have been; he weighed thirty pounds and the pig must have weighed six hundred. Even Vichy, at about a hundred pounds, would have been greatly overmatched.

Just then we heard the other trash can being knocked over. We only had two cans, so the pig's meal had to be nearly over.

The phone rang. It was our next-door neighbor.

"I think there's some sort of animal in your trash," she said. "I heard a can fall over and I think your dogs are barking." I thanked her for calling.

Then the phone rang again. It was the guy who lived behind us.

"Kendall, shut your damn dogs up! Nobody can sleep with that racket!"

And then it rang again. It was the yawning voice from the police station.

"You call 'bout the pig?" it asked.

"Yes. Is someone coming?"

"We needed to make sure it was a real call. We'll send a car."

I wondered if when someone called to report a murder whether they'd call back to make sure it was a real murder.

Our dining guest was now banging the two trash cans together and squealing.

"He's probably finished by now and wants some more," my wife said.

After a few more minutes there were no more sounds. It was nearly four now, and the police had not yet appeared. I told my wife to hold Orf while I went out to see what was going on.

I crept to the end of the house and peeked around the corner. Trash was all over the side yard and one can was smashed, but there was no pig! Orf and Vichy were still going wild inside, but evidently our friend had finished and taken off.

I flipped off my flashlight and turned to go back in the house. As I passed by our small Opel station wagon, only a dim silhouette in the poorly starlit night, it moved—and then it grunted.

Then I remembered the car was in the garage.

I turned the flashlight back on and aimed it at the grunt. There he was, three feet from me and coming my way!

Before I could decide whether to run or to pray, he was right next to me. Remember—this guy was as tall as my chest and I'm a fairly tall person. I could see my tombstone:

HERE LIES

GRANT KENDALL

(OR WHAT'S LEFT OF HIM)

MISTAKEN FOR A SLOP BUCKET

ON A DARK NIGHT

I was too young to die! There were so many things I hadn't done! (Now, a quarter century later, most of them are still not done.)

Then he made contact with me!

He pushed his head under my hand and began moving it from side to side. He wanted his head to be scratched! Thank goodness, he was a Gina, not a Sarah.

I scratched his head and stroked his ears. He moved up next to me and began rubbing against me, almost knocking me over. I called to my wife.

"Come on out here and take a look at this!"

She came forward very timidly. She is not very tall and he came nearly to her shoulders. After a little encouragement from me, she began petting him, too.

Then a pickup truck drove by.

"There he is!" came a shout from the truck.

It stopped, backed up and pulled in our driveway. A half-dozen people climbed out—three from the cab and three from the bed.

"I hope he din't bother you, mister," said one of the men. In the dark I couldn't tell how old he was, but his voice had a little age on it.

There were three other males and two females, but whether they were young or old I couldn't tell.

"Cyril, you been a bad boy!" scolded a female voice. The pig oinked and squealed and wiggled over toward her. "We been lookin' everywhere for you," she continued.

The whole group gathered around Cyril and cooed and petted on him. "We was sure worried, ol' boy," a male voice said.

The man who spoke first spoke again. "Somebody din't close his gate and he jest walked off. We been lookin' for him all night. We had to find him afore the kids got up in the mornin' and found out he was gone."

"Where do you live?" my wife asked.

"Jest down the road two-three miles," he answered, pointing off into the darkness. "We sure are glad to find ol' Cyril. He's a fine pig."

"What do you do with him?" my wife asked.

"Oh, he's our pet!" a female voice said proudly. "He's better'n any dog we ever had."

"How are you gonna get him home?" I asked.

"We'll jest walk him there. He'll foller us anywheres," the first voice replied. Then he said to some of his group, "Sammy and Wally, you start off with him and we'll be right behind you in the truck."

Two of the males—Sammy and Wally, I assumed—began walking off down the road. One of them said, "C'mon, Cyril. Let's go home."

Cyril oinked and snorted and trotted off after them.

"Cyril, you sure been naughty," Sammy or Wally said, as they ambled down the street.

The first voice spoke again. "Mister, I hope Cyril din't hurt nothin'."

"No, sir. No real harm done." But I unconsciously glanced over my shoulder toward the garbage cans.

"Jest what did he do?" the man asked.

"Nothing. Really," I insisted.

"Let me see that thing," he said, and took the flashlight from my hand. He shone it around the corner of the house.

"Oh, my goodness!" he exclaimed. "Look what Cyril done! Oh, mister, we sure are sorry. We'll fix everythin'!"

I tried to assure him that it wasn't necessary, that I was just glad that Cyril's family had found him.

The remaining four climbed back into the pickup's cab—it was a snug fit—and as they drove away after Sammy, Wally and Cyril, I heard the driver yell, "We'll be back and fix everythin'!"

It was after four-thirty now, and my wife and I crawled back in bed to try to get a little more sleep before we had to get up at six. She finally fell asleep around five, but I ended up getting up and studying. Sleep just wouldn't come.

She woke up at six, and we ate breakfast, made our lunches and got ready to leave. It was nearly six forty-five when the doorbell rang.

My wife answered it. It was the police.

"Where's the pig?" asked the officer.

She asked him where they'd been for the three and a half hours since we had called. She received no reply. She told him the pig had left, and then so did the police.

We left for school.

We got home around four-thirty that afternoon. As we turned into the driveway, I complained, "I've got Cyril's mess to clean up, and I don't think that one trash can is even usable anymore. I guess we'll have to buy a new one."

We went inside, and I changed into some mess-cleaning-up clothes and went back outside. I walked around the corner of the house and couldn't believe what I saw.

There was not a speck of trash anywhere to be seen. The trash can that had not been crushed was sitting neatly next to the garage, and next to it was a shiny new galvanized trash can, just like the one that had been smashed, which was nowhere to be seen.

I showed my wife. "He said they'd fix everything," she reminded me.

SPOT

The mare lay there. Uterine contractions had long since ceased, but the little—though "little" is hardly the word—foal still had his hindquarters in his dam.

This farm, in the Virginia countryside about thirty or forty miles from Washington, D.C., bred miniature horses. Or, rather, the miniature horses bred themselves. Each tiny stallion had his own harem in his own field. Each would spend the summer with his ladies and then be removed from them in the early fall.

The little mares were then on their own. The ones that were pregnant eventually foaled. They were left to do this in their own fields and not taken to the barn until the day after their foals arrived. Foaling was *au naturel*, and Mother Nature handled it pretty well, as a rule.

This mare, though, had evidently started the birthing process sometime overnight and had been unable to complete it. I was the farm's vet, and the owner called me about eight A.M. and reported the problem. "The foal's half out, the mare's not straining, and I can't pull it," he told me.

"Is the foal alive?" I asked.

"You bet," he replied. "He's waving those little front feet frantically."

I went there immediately. The little guy was bone dry and obviously not too pleased with his situation. He whinnied and thrashed, but still his rear stayed firmly within Mom.

The mare, in the meantime, was alive but worn out; she made minimal response to her baby's calls and efforts. I attempted to insert my hand around the foal and into the vagina, but there was no room and there was no natural lubricant. From all appearances, this birth had been going on for a *long* time.

I grabbed some lube from my trunk and applied it generously around the vulva and on my hands, but still I could not get a hand in. I tried to push the foal back into the mare a little, hoping to carry a little lube in that way, but he wouldn't budge. And he thought little of the maneuver.

It was apparent that we had the quintessential hip-lock. These aren't rare, but neither are they common; if detected early, a little rotation and/or manipulation alleviates the problem. But this one was *not* detected early.

One undesirable consequence of a hip-lock that goes on for a while is often a dead foal. If the foal does not get far enough out for his lungs to be able to expand, he can't breathe. The umbilicus frequently breaks, and all in all you have a sorry situation.

But this little guy had his chest well out, beyond the ribs, so breathing was possible. In fact, the more I fooled with him, the harder he worked at it. After a few minutes, he was almost panting.

We were getting nowhere, though, and I was at a loss as to what to do next. But then the little mare made the decision easy.

She died.

Immediately I grabbed my metal worming cup from the car and expressed into it about six ounces of colostrum from the mare's bag and set it aside.

At this point in my veterinary life I worked in a general large-animal practice. I had been unable to find employment in an exclusively equine practice, so I took the closest thing I could find. But I still had to do about thirty percent cattle and pigs. As I'm on record saying, pigs are okay, but cattle are only good when properly cooked. The cattle were proving important right now, however, because of some of the equipment I had to carry with me.

If a cow died on some remote farm, it was often necessary to determine the cause. It was impractical or, in many cases, impossible to transport her to a proper facility (laboratory or university), so field postmortems often had to be performed. For this purpose, my employer supplied me with a large, very sharp knife and a wicked-looking instrument that strongly resembled pruning shears but were, in reality, bone-cutters.

I got these tools out and rolled the mare up on her back, a maneuver singularly unappreciated by the foal. The owner helped steady the dead mare, and I used the knife to open her at the junction of her left hind leg and abdomen. I sliced down to the pelvis, then took the bone-cutters and severed the pelvic girdle through the ischium and pubis. (This is more easily written than accomplished.)

I thought this would allow enough extra movement to extricate the little guy, but still I could not budge him. I was beginning to think I'd picked up super glue instead of lube.

He was getting frantic now. I guess he'd decided that the time was well past when he should have been fully delivered; his owner was being severely battered by tiny front feet flying in all directions.

I took the knife and sliced open the area opposite the first incision and cut through the right pelvic bones as I had done with the left. Finally, as we pulled both of the mare's legs to the sides, we had a little space. With the owner straddling the corpse, holding the severed bones apart, I gave a prodigious tug to the colt, and out he came!

He lay there for a moment or two, perfectly still and just blinking. His right side was up, and on the point of the hip was a lesion about three inches in diameter and completely through the skin.

Then he began flopping and succeeded in flipping himself over. An identical lesion was on the left hip point. He had been pushed so hard by his mother that the contact points between his hips and her pelvis had literally shredded his hide.

But he was totally in the world now, and his needs had to be met, which meant he had to receive his colostrum. Normally I would pass a nasogastric tube in a neonate that was unable to nurse (for whatever reason), but the average neonate foal that I encountered generally weighed in the range of a hundred pounds and had nostrils suffi-ciently large to accept a tube. This fellow, however, probably weighed fifteen pounds, and there was no way I would be able to pass even my smallest tube through his teeny nostrils.

Allowing him to attempt to nurse was obviously the easiest choice. I had a lamb's nipple in the car, and my addiction to soft drinks meant that I always had a pop bottle. (Due to the fact that I mucked out my vehicles only semi-annually, I usually had around thirty pop bottles, actually.)

I poured the colostrum into a bottle, placed the nipple over the end and expressed a little into the colt's mouth. This was apparently what he had been waiting for his entire life; he glommed onto the nipple and eagerly sucked the colostrum down.

We medicated his hips and tried to help him up. The front end was willing, but the hindquarters were reluctant. We gave him a break, and I turned again to his lifeless dam to see what trauma may have been done to her in the dystocia.

The uterine wall had two large tears. This foal was not going to be born naturally, at least not out of this mare. There was just no space. Mother Nature would have culled them, but our intervention ended up halving the culling process.

The owner's wife had an upholstery shop on the farm. He said that's where the foal needed to be so he could have the frequent atten-tion he needed. He picked him up, and we put him in my car and drove to the shop.

His wife was a chunky woman who always seemed to be smiling, even when she wasn't. She was always surrounded by animals; the doors to the shop were always open in all kinds of weather, and animals of all description came and went at will.

There were at least a dozen dogs, from a very small Jack Russell to a very large you-name-it, and probably eight or nine cats. A very large sheep was usually there, as was a totally obnoxious goat. The pond in front of the shop sported dozens of ducks of various breeds, and they, too, frequented the inner recesses of the shop at will.

So when we delivered the little newcomer, the owner's wife was glad to see him. She placed some soft upholstering materials in a corner, and her husband placed the colt on them.

Immediately six or seven dogs began investigating the interloper. One, an aged Labrador who had had many litters, took especial interest; she began licking and nuzzling him, and in a minute was lying down beside him.

We retired to an old, partially re-covered couch, and I instructed the owners on getting some mare's milk replacer and a squeeze enema, and we talked over how to work with him to get him to stand.

After a short while I got up to leave, but before I went we walked around the corner to check on the foal again. Two-thirds of my directions ended up being useless; he was standing, still being licked by the Lab, and an enema was no longer necessary.

The owner got the milk replacer, and the little guy continued to take the bottle readily and frequently. We tended to the lesions on his hips and they healed quickly, but the hair came in white. His natural color was a grayish brown (I imagine it has a name, but if it's not bay, chestnut, or gray, I don't know what it's called), and these two baseball-sized white spots really stood out. Inevitably, he was named Spot.

Spot grew well as the foster child of the old Lab. He came and went with the dogs and other critters and, amazingly, seemed to become housebroken.

He ran with the dogs and played doggy games, although a little roughly for the smaller canines. By four months, he was off the bottle and onto dog food. I didn't think this was a good idea and convinced the owners to mix a little horse feed in with the dry dog food to try to get him onto a more suitable diet.

He had grown to the size of a middle-sized dog, maybe an Australian Shepherd. It was getting to the point where he should be with his own kind, I thought, so one day we took him to the field where he had been foaled. There were six or eight other mini-foals there, and it was natural, I thought, for him to want to be with them. But it never occurred to me that he had never looked into a mirror. He didn't know that he looked like them.

We turned him in with the other little horses, and he indicated, loudly and for all to hear, that this was not the course he wished to take with his life. I left, listening to him bellow, and didn't return for several days.

On my next visit to the farm, the dogs, as usual, came bounding and barking to greet me. And with them was Spot.

"He just doesn't think he's a horse," the owner's wife explained. "He was so unhappy."

I went off with the owner to attend to things, and as I was finishing, his wife was motoring out the drive in her van. She waved as she passed us, and in the back a half-dozen various and sundry dogs bounced around. And right in the middle, watching us out of the rear window, was Spot!

I looked at the owner.

"He loves to go to town," he explained.

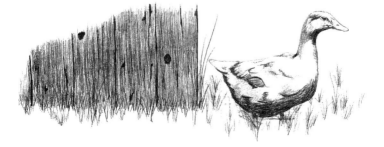

BAA

I know very little about sheep. In school I learned very little about sheep. I vaguely recall that they have their own special diseases, in addition to the general problems common to all ruminants. I won't swear to any of this, though.

One of the reasons for my profound lack of sheep knowledge is that I went to vet school in a state that had very few sheep. *Very* few. We were told somewhere along the line that there were more sheep in a modest-sized flock in Wyoming or Montana than in our whole state.

Another reason, which I guess ties right in with the first reason, is that no one on the faculty knew anything about sheep.

There was one faculty member, however—Dr. David Crone— who came from out west (Utah, I believe) and had actually *seen* sheep, which put him miles ahead of most of his peers at the school. He hadn't ever really worked with them, but at least the vet school he attended taught sheep medicine.

One day in our Large Animal Medicine course, our regular teacher, Dr. John Emery, announced that we would be instructed in General Sheep that day, and that Dr. Crone would do it. We were then exposed to nearly fifty minutes on the subject, the gist of which was: Sheep exist.

Perhaps some of my classmates gleaned a little more knowledge on the subject that day than I did, but I doubt it. Ninety-five percent of them went into pet practice; one or two students went into cattle practice, one into swine, and the other two of us chose horses. I imagine there was a question concerning sheep on an exam somewhere, but I can't say for sure. If there was, I missed it.

About a month after graduation, I learned a little about sheep. Virginia, of course, was (is) not renowned sheep-producing country, but one morning I received a hysterical phone call from a woman with a heavy Eastern European accent.

"Da sheepa's bin hurted!" she cried. "Come kvick!"

I tried to get further details but couldn't. I speak rather rapidly and she couldn't understand me, and the more I questioned her the more excited she became. With the excitement came a thickening of her accent and a lapse into her native tongue. I was able to get an address, though, and I hurried there.

Da sheepa had indeed bin hurted. I found her husband and son with about a dozen dead and dying sheep. Evidently a pack of dogs had gotten into the small flock overnight. And, although the sheep were covered with blood, they weren't dying from their wounds. They were dying from shock.

This is what I learned that day:

1. Sheep have *very* thin skin.
2. When the thin skin is broken, they bleed.
3. Sheep are basically white outside (I actually knew this before).
4. Sheep blood is red (I suspected this).
5. When the red blood gets on the white sheep, it makes a horrible mess.
6. Sheep evidently go into shock easily and readily and die more easily and more readily.

7. After speaking with the husband, the wife's command of the
   English language took on 'enry 'iggins-like proportions.

For about five years, that's where my sheep knowledge
remained. I moved to central Kentucky and set up my present equine
practice and reduced my chances of contact with the ovine species to
near zero. I thought.

One of my clients is Glenraven Farm, a family-run operation
that usually has about twenty-five mares, either boarded or farm-
owned. Now they have an employee, but back then their kids were in
their teens and everything was done by the family.

I drove in one day and Cheryl Glendon, the thirteen-year-old
daughter, greeted me at the barn.

"Come see what we have," she enthused.

I followed her to the foaling stall, and she proudly showed me
two lambs.

"They're for the State Fair," she said, beaming. "Rodney and I
are gonna raise and show them."

Rodney was fourteen and extremely nonagricultural—he
washed his hands immediately after handling a horse, which meant he
washed several times a day—but that was not my problem. I pictured
Susan Glendon, known to the kids as "Mom," as having seen this as a
way to pique Rodney's interest in things biological. It wouldn't work;
I knew that and Roger ("Dad") knew that, and I strongly suspect
Susan knew that, too, but hope springs eternal, as they say. Rodney
liked rock music and cars, and probably the only biological thing
that would pique any of his fourteen-year-old interest would be a
fourteen-year-old girl.

But that wasn't my problem, either. I thought.

The lambs, named Baa (Cheryl's) and Bo (Rodney's), were little,
cute and being bottle-fed. Shortly they became bigger, less cute and
real food–fed. They were being coddled and groomed and allowed to
graze for a short period each day, but basically their home was the
foaling stall. It was late June and the stall wouldn't be needed again
until late January, and as the State Fair was held at the end of August,
they would be long gone by then.

The doors to all the stalls at Glenraven were inward-swinging, and so that they would swing freely over the stall bedding, the bottoms were about four inches above the floor. To prevent horses from accidentally injuring their legs by sticking them through this four-inch gap, each doorway was fitted with a removable board that fit into slots on either side of the opening, thereby eliminating the gap and any danger.

This is where I learned more about sheep. Rodney did not replace the board in the foaling stall one day after grooming his lamb. I imagine he was in a hurry to wash his hands.

Baa, Cheryl's lamb (of course), lay down right at the doorway and went into full lateral recumbency. Both hind legs evidently extended through the gap and into the barn aisle.

Enter a new character—Flog, the Glendons' dog. Flog was of indeterminate ancestry but definite size—about seventy-five or eighty pounds. He had shown mild interest in the sheep since their arrival but nothing more.

Susan ("Mom") came to the barn, and Flog was with her. Flog saw these things extending under the foaling stall door and probably didn't stop to consider his actions. He ran to them, picked one up and began carrying it off. He didn't get far, however, as the attached lamb remained on the other side of the door, but he did carry it far enough for Susan to hear a decided "Crack!" followed by a pathetic bleat.

Susan called me on my mobile phone. "Grant, one of the lambs has a broken leg! Please come and do something!" I now had another sheep patient.

I went directly to Glenraven. I wasn't at all sure what to do, but when I heard the whole story I suggested shooting Rodney and Flog. Cheryl agreed to shoot Rodney, but Susan vetoed shooting either one of them.

I examined the leg. It was the left hind, and Susan's diagnosis was correct—it was broken, snapped in mid-cannon.

I explained to them the costs of X rays, the possible need to pin or plate the bone, the recovery period, the good chance that he wouldn't be ready for the fair, etc. I suggested that a leg-of-lamb dinner might be the appropriate remedy to the problem.

By this time, Roger and Rodney had arrived, and the four of them stepped into the feed room for a family conference while I straightened up things in my trunk. I could hear very little of what was being said, only the occasional "We're not going to eat Baa!" as Cheryl raised her voice.

They came back out after several minutes. Cheryl was wiping away tears and glaring at Rodney. "Save the lamb," Roger said, shaking his head.

I was starting to get out my radiograph machine when Roger added, "But it can't cost much."

I put the machine back in the car. "How 'bout we put a cast on there for a few weeks and see what we end up with?" I asked.

They agreed to try it.

By lining up the two ends of the bone manually—I had no idea how well they were really aligned—and having Roger and Rodney hold Baa down, I applied a plaster cast. It was a warm day, so the plaster set up quickly.

When we finished, Roger and I helped Baa to his feet and Rodney went to wash his hands. Baa stood there looking back at his leg, which he held a little off the stall floor. After maybe thirty seconds he gingerly placed the foot down and hazarded a few steps. At first he dragged it along, but shortly he began to use it a little.

I told them to eliminate his grazing time and just keep him in the stall, and I'd check him each time I came to the farm. The breeding season was over, so I was there only once or twice a week.

Three or four days later I looked in on Baa. He appeared to be fine, but I wanted to check him anyway. We laid him down; I pinched him between the toes and he responded by pulling back. This indicated that there was feeling in the leg and that the cast was not too tight.

After nearly four weeks, Cheryl asked, "When will you take the cast off?"

Good question. Baa was young and young bones heal rapidly, assuming we had gotten the two ends together properly. And the fair was in a little less than a month.

"I guess we'll do it right now," I said. And we did.

The leg was thinner than it had been, of course, but there was no palpable fracture anymore. We let him up and told him to walk on it, but he ignored us. He stood there, holding the leg about three inches off the ground.

I popped him on the rear with the palm of my hand; he bleated and scooted across the stall—on three legs. We tried lifting another leg. He would balance on us, or if we let go quickly, he would fall. But he wouldn't put the once-broken leg down.

By manipulation I could see that he had both motor and sensory function to the leg, so we decided to see how he'd do for a couple of days.

Two days later he was still three-legged. Cheryl pointed out how unlikely it would be for a three-legged lamb to do any good at the State Fair.

I called some other vets in the area. There are a couple of large-animal practitioners around here, but their knowledge of sheep was not much greater than mine, and neither of them had ever mended a broken ovine leg.

Then I called a small-animal friend and asked her how she managed a dog or cat that wouldn't use a leg. She suggested that we tie up another leg—the other hind leg or the opposite front leg—and see if that wouldn't force him to use it.

Tying up a sheep's leg, as it turned out, was easier for her to suggest than it was for us to do. Finally, however, with yards of gauze and tape, we had Baa's right hind leg rendered unusable.

He wouldn't get up. We picked him up and tried to get him to balance, but he wouldn't.

He put his front legs out and sat there like a dog, his two hind legs, for different reasons, unusable. Several further attempts yielded the same results.

Back to the drawing board. We released the right hind leg and began to work on the right *front* leg. It, too, required miles of gauze and tape, but in time we had it in a makeshift sling.

But still no success. The only difference was that now Baa couldn't even dog-sit. He lay there looking pathetic. Sheep, by the way, are very good at looking pathetic.

This was becoming a challenge! We undid the leg, and after a few minutes Baa got up, still three-legged.

I told the Glendons I'd be back, but first I had to check with some more people. I had no idea who; I was just trying to buy time to see if I could come up with *something*.

I went home and called my old alma mater and asked to speak with Dr. Crone.

"We have no Dr. Crone here," came the switchboard operator's reply.

Well, it *had* been more than seven years. I guess he was entitled to go elsewhere to work, even though it wasn't very considerate of him.

"Then let me speak with Dr. Emery," I said. I knew *he* was still there—he was an institution at the institution—and maybe he had come across a sheep since I had last seen him.

"Grant, great to hear from you!" he greeted me. He's a great guy even if he does like cows.

I explained the problem to him. He had no ideas at all.

"Who would?" I asked.

"Try Bob Wildman at Colorado State. That's sheep country."

So I tried Bob Wildman. This guy wrote the book on sheep, and he had actually seen *two* broken-legged lambs that the owners wanted to save, but he had not seen this problem. Struck out again.

That evening I received a call from RiverEdge Farm. A mare was colicking. This was something I knew a little about, so I went right out there.

RiverEdge only had eight mares; it was primarily a cattle farm. And management knew better than to have me doctor their cows.

When I got there I tended to the mare—a little gas, nothing serious—and as I was packing up to leave I heard a decidedly bovine bellow from the other end of the barn.

"What's that?" I asked.

"Oh, that's one of the bulls. He hurt his foot and wouldn't walk on it. Doc Walton found a big ol' rock wedged between his toes and he's just stayin' in for a couple of days 'til it's not so sore."

"He had a rock stuck between his toes and couldn't walk?"

"Well, yeah, he could walk, but he didn't want to. It hurt. He was hoppin' around out there three-legged."

If I had been a cartoon character, a light bulb would have appeared over my head.

When I got home I visited my son's toy chest, and the next morning I went to see Baa, armed with two marbles, one regular-sized and one big.

We flopped him on his side once more and I stuck the regular marble tightly between the toes of his right hind foot. He didn't think much of this procedure. Then I wrapped the foot with tape—lots of tape—to keep the marble in place. Messrs. Johnson & Johnson were probably getting very fond of me after this and the leg-tying-up fiasco of the previous day.

We got him up, and he staggered off on three legs. The right foot was obviously uncomfortable but not uncomfortable enough to make him put the left foot down—it was still a few inches above the ground.

Down he went again. I removed all the tape and the marble and wedged in the larger marble and taped *it* in place. I made a mental note to see what Johnson & Johnson shares were selling for.

We got him up again. He stepped down on the marbled foot and immediately jerked it up. This gave him two hind feet off the ground at the same time, a position most sheep can't hold for long, and he fell.

We got him up again. This time, as he put pressure on the marble, he picked the foot up a little more carefully and placed the left foot on the ground!

He was still off balance so he fell once more, but we got him up again. This time he was a little more deliberate in all his actions and he was able to stay upright. He began walking very slowly, moving each hind leg very gradually and carefully, one because it was painful and one because he probably *thought* it was painful.

I left then. I had a living to make and hadn't charged for any of Baa's treatment, not even for the tape. I called that evening. Yes, he had been up several times, and yes, he had walked on the left leg.

I went back two days later and he was still using both legs. I figured we had to get the marble out before anything serious happened to the right foot.

"What happens if he doesn't walk on the broken leg again?" Cheryl asked.

"Oh, he will!" I stated confidently. We had been taught in school never to say anything like that, but I think most of us do it every once in a while. And we're right often enough to get by with it. Usually, though, we have an inkling of what we're talking about.

The gods do smile down sometimes. We got the marble out and put Baa back on his feet. He stood there on all four. Cheryl gave him a little push and he walked off—hesitatingly—using all four legs.

And the problem was over. Baa used the broken leg better each day, and by State Fair time you couldn't tell he had ever had a problem. Even with restriction and injury, he had far surpassed Bo in size and appearance. Maybe the extra TLC he received helped. Bo, however, had been groomed with cleaner hands.

I know nothing about sheep classes and judging and I want to maintain my knowledge at that level, so I have no idea how "good" these two lambs were. But Baa must have been okay; he was judged the second best in the fair.

It's many years later now. Cheryl and Rodney are grown and Flog long ago went to the Great Kennel in the Sky. Cheryl breeds and shows dogs and still enjoys working with her parents on the farm when time allows. Rodney is a studio musician in Atlanta—some kind of horn, I think. I've often wondered if he washes his hands after each session.

"CAT"

It was about seven-thirty when we pulled into the driveway. We had been to visit my grandmother, who was residing in a retirement home, one of those places where all the residents' needs are attended to.

Grandma wasted nothing. Invariably when we visited, she would have a bag of things for us that were no longer needed or had been discarded by her co-inhabitants of the home. We would come home with half-used pieces of paper ("scratch paper"), a week's worth of rubber bands from the newspapers delivered there, old magazines, calibrated medicine cups, one or two unused Band-Aids, etc.

And especially she did not waste food. Anything not eaten that day was gathered up by Grandma and saved for us. We only visited once a week, and I know it must have been agony for her to not be able to give us all of the leftovers from the other days.

Please understand. She didn't want us to eat these scraps; they were for our pets—two dogs and a cat. And the animals appreciated her thoughtfulness.

On this particular evening, they had had salmon croquettes for dinner at the retirement home. Evidently they didn't go over too well, because Grandma had a bag of about a dozen for us. It was late February and very chilly, so we had the car windows up and the heater on as we drove home. Our goody bag, in the heat and close quarters, began to smell increasingly fishy.

Then, as we opened the doors to get out at home, we unleashed all of this trapped, warm, salmon-soaked air into the cool winter evening. Anyone within two miles probably thought that the area was being attacked by a force armed with fish sticks.

Within seconds of the time we stepped from the car, a cat ran up to us, vocally expressing itself to the brown paper bag my wife was holding. Neither of us had ever seen this animal before; it was a typically marked grey-and-white and singularly unattractive. That is to say, ugly. It was, however, hungry.

"Give her one of those things," I said to my wife.

She dropped a croquette on the ground. The cat almost inhaled it. My wife put down two or three more with the same result.

The cat followed us to the door. "Give it some more," I suggested. We ended up emptying the whole contents of the bag, and the cat ate every croquette.

I guess it was no surprise when the cat greeted me the next morning as I headed toward the barn. It wanted to know where the salmon was this morning.

The barn is a good hike from the house; on rainy or particularly cold days, or if I was heading off somewhere afterwards, I would drive there. This morning I was going into town, so I got into the car. To my astonishment, the cat jumped in with me. The fact that the car still smelled like a fish factory may have been an incentive.

In my experience, before and since, cats are *not* good car travelers. I don't know if it's the motion or the noise or what, but they don't like it. Our house cat, for example, would stand in my lap with her front feet on my chest and her nose on mine and howl until such time as the ride was over. This cat, however, just sat on the seat beside me and rode quietly.

I got out at the barn; the cat got out at the barn. I fed the horses, turned them out and did all that I needed to do, then went back to the car. The cat went with me. It seemed as if I had acquired a friend.

We needed a barn cat. Badly. The house cat did not think a barn was a suitable environment and I had put off getting a kitten for fear of its safety. We had mice, which were no threat, but we had at least one rat. The first time I saw it I thought a foal had gotten into the feed room, except that we didn't have any foals that big at the time. And, I figured, if we had one rat we probably had two.

I had put out rat poison, but even though I had had good success in the past with the stuff, it did not seem to affect the present problem.

I took the new cat and closed it in the feed room. I would buy some cat food in town and make the barn a desirable place, and maybe it would stay.

When I returned with the cat food, the cat was still there. I told my wife of our new resident. We decided to make sure it was going to stay and then we'd have it spayed or neutered, whichever was applicable.

That afternoon the cat was still there at the barn, and a good portion of the cat food I had put out that morning was gone. I picked the animal up and checked to see if the future held a spaying or a neutering. It was a female.

The next morning she greeted me at the door again. I walked to the barn this time and she was right at my heels. When I reached the barn, in the aisle was about a third of a rat.

Every morning she would greet me at the door and walk or ride with me to the barn. Over a period of ten days or so, any evidence of a rodent problem disappeared.

She still hadn't been named. I had just been calling her Cat and she hadn't seemed to mind, so Cat she became. It was now pretty apparent that she was going to stay, so the time had come to have her spayed.

But a problem arose. She was very pregnant. Oh well, I thought, we'll wean the kittens and then have it done. We'll just hope for a small litter.

Cat's interaction with our dogs was unremarkable. At this time, we still had Orf, who was now very old and had been around cats all his life, and a Fox Terrier named Gypsy, who had also been raised with a cat, and they paid no attention to her. Or she to them.

But the relationship with Annie, the house cat, was something altogether different.

Annie needs an introduction. She was about three years old then and had been an only cat all her life. Although a house cat, she did go outside, but when nature called she would come back to the house, climb the screen door and howl at the top of her lungs until someone let her in. Then she would run as fast as she could to her sand box, relieve herself, then return to the door and ask to be let out in the same manner in which she had requested entrance.

One day, after Cat had been with us a few days, she and Annie met in the front yard. My wife saw the whole thing. They saw each other from about four feet and for the next ten minutes they scrunched down on their bellies and hissed and spat at each other. Neither attacked nor retreated. Finally my wife picked up Annie and brought her in.

And that was the extent of their relationship. Whenever they happened across each other, they would scrunch down and hiss and spit until one was carried away. Then the other would continue as if nothing had ever happened in the first place.

Back to Cat's pregnancy. About two weeks after I noticed her condition, she gave birth to four very healthy kittens. Okay, we'd find a home for them, give her a week or so for her milk to dry up and then have her spayed.

She was a good provider for her children. One day, when they were about three weeks old, I found the four kittens growling and fighting over a rabbit carcass, evidently supplied by mother. It must have been quite a battle; the rabbit was every bit as big as Cat.

And as time passed I found remnants of others of Cat's hunts—mice, birds, another rabbit. The cats weren't hungry—there was free-choice cat food at all times—but I guess Cat was a hunter at heart.

We found homes for all four kittens by the time they were six weeks old. A couple of weeks after the last one left, I took Cat into the local small animal vet. His first comment on seeing her was, "Boy, is that an ugly cat!" Then he checked her over and said, "Grant, are you sure you want to spay her now?"

"Sure. Why?"

"She's pregnant. She's about two weeks away."

Her kittens were about eight weeks old. I had long since forgotten most of what I had learned about cats in school, but my friend explained that frequently they do have a "foal heat." Obviously Cat had had one.

Well, I decided to let her have *this* litter and then spay her.

She had four more kittens this time and fed them as she had fed the first group, with rabbits, rodents, birds—anything Cat could catch.

Again we found homes for the kittens, but it was a little more of a challenge this time. When the last one left at about eight weeks, I took her in without waiting for her milk to go totally.

"Grant, I think she's pregnant again."

Back to the barn she went, surgery being put off once more. And true to form, she delivered four more very vigorous offspring. And true to form, she fed them from nature's table—for a while.

One morning, though, when the kittens were a month old, I found them fighting over a chicken! A huge chicken. It was twice the size of Cat.

Our area is not one known for wild chickens, but the people two farms down the road, about a quarter mile, kept several chickens for the eggs. I suspected they had one fewer now.

And a few days later, they had two fewer. Maybe the first one had been sick or suicidal, but it's unlikely the flock would contain two such as that. Cat was obviously killing these birds that were much bigger than she was.

The neighbors kept their chickens in a coop. I guess there was no problem in Cat gaining entrance, but I couldn't imagine how she got the huge birds out. But she did.

A few days later, while I was out front mowing along the road, my chicken-owning neighbor pulled over and stopped.

"Hi, Mr. Clark," I said.

"Howdy, Doc. You seen any foxes? I think we got foxes."

"Foxes? No, I haven't seen any. Why?"

"I've lost three or four hens in the last week."

"I'll be darned."

I guess Cat decided these were easier prey for her, all neatly penned up as they were. I talked to her about it, and although she was always an attentive listener, I don't think she was convinced enough to change her evil ways.

This third batch of four kittens was a real test for us to find homes for. We had used up all of our friends on the two earlier litters; this time we put little notices up in places like markets, feed stores and the vet's office, among others. In time, though, all four were in the hands of loving new owners, and Cat and I were off to the clinic again.

"Guess what?" the vet said.

"No kidding," I said.

"And she's sitting on 'go' now. I bet she'll have them within three or four days."

I should have taken his bet. It was a week, but she had four again.

The first meal I found her delivering to this family was Mr. Clark's rooster. It was immense.

When the kittens were a month old, I decided that early weaning was indicated. Once more Cat and I went to the vet.

This time the surgery was performed. It had to be—I was beginning to worry about the foals. Any cat that could tackle that rooster wouldn't find much of a problem with a little horse.

I picked her up later that afternoon. He told me that she had been pregnant again, but only about three weeks along. A study in fertility.

But the hunting stopped. At least I saw no more evidence of her forays. Mr. Clark reported no further lost chickens. (He had been furious over his rooster.)

The last litter of four was tough. We ran newspaper ads, we announced "free kittens" on the radio, we went up to total strangers and said, "Please!" Finally they were gone.

Cat still patrols the barn, and there hasn't been a rodent problem in several years now. She still meets me at the door in the mornings. She's still ugly.

(In case anyone thinks Mr. Clark suffered unfair losses, I paid him for his chickens. I had no idea what they cost and I didn't have the courage to tell him that I knew what happened to them, so I mailed him a twenty-dollar bill anonymously.)

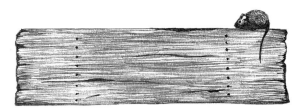

DAISY

I enjoy waterfowl. We have a small pond on our small farm, and now we have around three dozen resident ducks and geese, but it wasn't always so well populated.

When we first bought the farm, the pond had no birds, not even passersby. Wild ducks and geese would fly overhead going or coming to or from wherever they came from or went to, but none would ever stop and visit.

I'd be outside doing something and a flock would pass over and I'd yell, "Hey, guys, here's a pond!" I'd point to it so they would know where it was. "You're welcome to stay here! Or just stop over! I like you!" I'd bellow as they disappeared over the horizon.

But they wouldn't listen. They'd just keep on flapping and flying, without even a quack of acknowledgment.

One spring day, after we'd been on the farm about a year and a half, I stopped in the local feed store to place an order, and they had a whole batch of baby mallards sitting there for sale. They were only $3.95 a pair, and how wrong could you go for $3.95?

I bought a pair. They were little—both of them fit in one hand—and very fuzzy. My knowledge of duck care was extremely limited, and I said as much to the feed store employee who took my money.

"Shoot, ain't nothin' to it," he informed me. "Just feed 'em."

"Feed 'em what?" And he sold me a fifty-pound sack of poultry starter ration.

"How much do I give them?" I queried.

"Oh, just put out a panful and keep it in front of 'em—sorta free choice."

Rough mental calculations told me that fifty pounds of starter feed would last two ducklings somewhere in the neighborhood of forever, but they had to eat, so I loaded up and headed home.

My wife and kids were delighted to see the ducklings, but my wife's pleasure waned a little when I told her we'd be keeping them in the bathtub until they got a little bigger. I just couldn't see putting anything that small out in the world on their own.

"I like to take baths," she protested.

"We have two bathrooms. You can just shower for a little while," I explained.

"*I like to take baths!*" she reiterated, but finally consented, albeit grudgingly.

Bathtub bottoms slope toward the drain end, of course, so they will empty efficiently when the plug is pulled. We ran enough water into the tub to fill it about halfway up the sloping bottom; in the upper end we placed a pie pan filled with starter ration.

Over the next couple of weeks we learned a great deal about ducks, mainly:

1. Ducks have atrocious table manners.
2. Ducks eat what seems to be forty times their own body weight daily.

3. Ducks' intestinal tracts convert the feed intake into roughly three times as much output. We had to drain and wash out the tub twice a day.

But they grew. Anything that ate that much *had* to grow. After what my wife called an eternity (the dictionary defines *eternity* as "endless time"; she defined it as being closer to two weeks), the ducklings' fuzz began turning to identifiable feathers. The decision was made to take them to the pond.

By this time these were well-tamed ducks. The kids had named them Bo and Daisy, with the hope that one would eventually prove to be a boy (Bo) and the other a girl (Daisy). They had been carried around the house or otherwise handled several times a day and had lost whatever innate fear of humans they may have had.

The four of us gathered up Bo, Daisy and the feed pan and toted them down to the pond, which was only about forty yards from the house. We set them down on the bank of what to them, at their sizes, must have looked like an ocean, even though it was only about a hundred feet wide. They just stood there for several minutes, until finally I patted them on their rears and scooted them into the water.

This was great! Their swimming in the shallow bathtub had been limited, but here they could splash and dive and zoom and zig and zag and do amazing water things they had never been able to do before.

We watched them for ten or fifteen minutes, then I said, "Well, they look as if they like it. Let's leave them." And we headed back to the house.

My wife went immediately to scrub down the tub, mumbling something about a three-hour bath.

I sat down in the family room to watch TV with the kids, but within two or three minutes we heard a small clicking sound coming from the back door.

It was Daisy and Bo! They had hopped up the step and were pecking at the glass door. My son opened the door, and they hopped over the threshold and came on in. They waddled straight to the bathroom door, which was closed, and sat there.

I stuck my head in the bathroom. "Move over," I said to my wife, "you have company." She wasn't amused.

It was pretty obvious that Bo and Daisy had enjoyed their little outing, but now they wanted to return to their natural habitat, i.e., the bathtub. The kids and I tried to explain to them where they really belonged as we took them back to the pond.

They came back three more times and we returned them to nature three more times. The last time I got out a large plastic pet carrier and put them in it with some feed and water and placed the whole thing on the pond bank. After spending the night there, they finally accepted the fact that they were no longer house ducks.

Bo and Daisy did well. They grew over the summer and turned into real mallards. Neither turned out to be a boy, though, but Bo was still a fine name for a girl.

Later, in the fall, we had visits from wild ducks. I assume they saw Bo and Daisy and realized the pond was okay. Some mornings there would be a hundred ducks on it, mostly mallards but a few other kinds as well. And even a few Canadian geese stopped by later in the year.

Our starter ration had run out, finally, and I had begun tossing them a little shell corn once or twice a day. The layovers scattered when I appeared to toss the corn, but as soon as I retreated they would return to partake of the feast.

But they'd always move on. Sometimes a group would stay for a few days or just a night, but sooner or later they'd continue their flights southward. I began wondering if Bo and Daisy would one day succumb to this natural phenomenon. Instinct is a powerful thing.

And, sure enough, one evening I couldn't find Bo. The large flock of mallards that had been there that morning was gone, and the only duck on the pond was Daisy.

She was not pleased. She was quacking loudly and swimming in circles, and after several days of this I began to think she was lonely. She had been much tamer than Bo and would come right up to me each time I appeared. She began following me to the barn in the mornings, sometimes right alongside Cat, and I would give her her corn there.

In time she made her home in a stall. She'd go to the pond occasionally, but she'd always fly back to the barn when she saw me go there.

One of my clients had a pond on which he and his wife kept several Pekins, the large white ducks after which Donald was undoubtedly patterned. These ducks would sometimes come to their barn, and one day when I was there I mentioned Daisy.

"She's an only duck," I told them, "and really seems to be lonely. I guess I'll have to buy a couple more ducklings next spring."

"Maybe we can help you," said my client. "One of our drakes is sort of an outcast. The other ducks chase him away all the time. Do you want him?"

"Yeah, that would be great."

They said they'd try to catch him when he came to the barn again.

A few days later they called. "Come get your duck," my client's wife said. "Bring something to put him in."

I took the pet carrier out there, and after ten minutes of trying to corner him in the stall they'd trapped him in—ducks have sharp claws, by the way—we finally succeeded in getting him into the carrier. He was angry!

I took him home and turned him loose at the barn, which was where Daisy met us. She took one look at him and took off for the pond! It was *not* love at first sight.

The kids named the new duck Scrooge. He hung around the barn all the time, and Daisy would meet me there, eat her corn and leave whenever she saw him.

One day I closed Scrooge in a stall. When Daisy came for her meal, I picked her up and put her in there, too. "Make friends," I told them.

They sat there in opposite corners of the stall, staring at each other. Neither moved. I put some water in the center of the stall in a horse ground-feeder and spread a little corn around it.

"If you guys are gonna eat and drink, you'll have to meet halfway to do it," I said, and went back to the house.

Later that evening I walked back to the barn to look in on them. It didn't appear as if either had moved.

"Boy, are you guys silly," I said, and went back and went to bed.

The next morning, however, the corn was gone and Scrooge and Daisy were both drinking from the feeder, side by side.

"That's better," I told them. "Now get out of here and be friends."

And they did. All winter they were inseparable. The pond froze, but that was not a problem to them—they had their barn.

One morning in the spring Scrooge greeted me at the barn, but Daisy was not with him. It wasn't the time of year when she might fly off, but it was the time, as was *any* time, when a hungry predator may have gotten her. That worried me, but I couldn't do anything about it.

A few days later my son asked me where Daisy was. I said I hadn't seen her in a while, but then my daughter said, "She's out front. I saw her there last night."

"Where?"

"Out in the front yard, just walking around pecking at the ground."

I asked her to show me, and she pointed out the front door. "There," she said. "That's the front yard."

But there was no Daisy there. I didn't want to disbelieve a six-year-old, but Daisy hadn't showed up for her corn for at least four days. She was gone.

The next evening I was catching up on some of the seemingly endless reading that is required to stay abreast of things in the veterinary world when my daughter came to my office door.

"Daddy, Daisy's out front again."

"Oh, baby, you know she's not."

"Yes, she is!" She frowned and stomped her foot.

I glared. "Show me."

She was right. Daisy was out there, pecking around in the grass. I went out to see her and she scooted under a very large boxwood, which had gotten that way because I always put off trimming it. (I have always felt that plant scientists should develop self-trimming bushes and self-mowing grass.)

I got down on my hands and knees and looked under the bush. There she was, sitting on a nest! I couldn't tell how many eggs there were, but it didn't matter. From then on 'til hatching I gave her a little corn under the bush each day.

One day when Daisy was seen out in the yard, we counted her eggs. There were twenty-six!

It seemed like months—but it was really only weeks—until they hatched. Two of the eggs didn't make it, but twenty-four of them did.

They were a strange lot. Some looked like little mallards and some were totally yellow, like baby Pekins. But most had varying shades and amounts of black and yellow, as they were a blend of their two parents.

Nature's attrition set in and two of the ducklings died, but by that summer the pond was populated by two dozen ducks—the proud parents and their twenty-two children. That fall the migrators would drop in for visits but would fly on, and none of ours would leave. I often wondered if Bo was ever among the visitors.

That was more than fifteen years ago. Daisy and Scrooge eventually disappeared—I guess they knew when their times had come and went to wherever ducks go at that time—but their legacy lives on. All those ducks out there now are their descendants.

MULES

Tom Ball is a horse trader. It's a hard way to make a living and very few can do it, but Tom is successful at it. He doesn't live high on the hog from it, but then Tom's tastes are rather simple. He feeds and houses his family and pays his bills. That's more than a lot of folks can manage.

The thing I like best about Tom Ball is that last attribute: bill paying. He insists on paying for everything he can the minute it's done. He won't buy new furniture or clothes unless he has the cash in hand to pay for it when he gets it.

"Cash in hand" is the key phrase here. Tom doesn't have a checking account. "I had one once and *never* knew how much money I had," he explained to me one day.

He'll drive a truck forever, and when he does finally get rid of it, he pays cash for the next one, which is not always new. The same goes for his wife's car. With proper care—and he does give them that—he figures he can get ten years out of a car. With the amount his wife drives, that's probably fewer than 70,000 miles.

Given his choice, I suspect Tom would like to pay for his electricity and water the same way. Watch an evening of TV, give the electric company a dollar or so. Take a bath, pay the water company. Unfortunately for him, they don't work that way.

It doesn't matter how much work I do for him, I have the cash in my hand before I leave the farm. He insists on a receipt, from me and from everyone he deals with. "You *got* to have records," he says.

Tom has run up some healthy bills at times. He sells a lot of horses at the local stockyards, and they all must have Coggins tests run on them before they can be shipped in. Usually he has maybe five or six to test, but once he received a truckload of animals from goodness knows where. There were twenty-two of them shipped in all at one time, and they all needed Coggins tests. He paid me on the spot—$330 in fives and tens.

Drawing blood for the tests is especially fun—considering the horses Tom gets in. Many of them are close to wild, so the experience is a true test of our fitness. But we always get it done.

Tom also buys horses from the stockyards. If he sees something that he feels he can sell privately for a profit, he'll bring it home. Once he bought an aged Thoroughbred mare that hadn't been in foal for a couple of years, but he thought she was in good enough shape to give her another chance. He bought her for $300 and talked the seller into giving him her registration certificate.

"My vet said she'd never have another foal," the guy had said. Maybe he was right, but it didn't matter. Her two-year-old later that year won over $300,000, and Tom sold her, not bred, for $3,500 to a man who wanted to see if *his* vet could accomplish anything with her.

That kind of profit was rare, but he'd frequently buy $50 and $70 ponies, keep them for a few weeks and then sell them to doting parents for $250 to $300. Profits usually weren't very large, but he'd make $100 on fifteen to twenty transactions a month, and the result was a decent living.

One day Tom called me out to look at a little mare he had bought a few days earlier at the stockyards. She had bumped an eye on something, and it was swollen shut. I found no damage to the eye itself, so we didn't do any treatment.

The mare was small, a little more than fourteen hands and about 650 pounds. She was kind of a mousy light bay but well made, with a kind disposition.

"Got a buyer for her yet?" I asked.

"Not yet. Might keep her for Vickie. She's been wantin' a horse of her own." Vickie was Tom's only child. I guess she was about eleven then.

Vickie named the little mare Queenie and began riding her. The next time I was there—maybe two weeks later—I noticed that Queenie had gained considerable weight.

"Tom, you're gonna founder her if you don't watch how much you're feeding," I warned.

"Doc, she's only gettin' a handful once a day, but she sure is blossomin'."

"Well, watch her closely." And I didn't think any more of it.

Tom's farm is not far from mine—three or four miles—and I often pass it as I'm going or coming. One morning about two weeks later, I left home early to tend a sick foal that had taken a turn for the worse overnight, and my route took me by Tom's place.

Queenie's paddock was one of about one and a half acres next to the road, right in front of the house. As I passed by I saw her lying down, which is, of course, permitted, but as I glanced a second time I saw what looked like a large trash bag behind her.

I turned in, drove to the house and got Tom.

"I think I know why Queenie's gotten so round," I told him.

"You stopped here at six-thirty in the morning to tell me that?"

"She was in foal," I said.

"What do you mean *was?*"

"Come see."

He called his wife and daughter and told them to get dressed and come out to see Queenie. Then he and I went on out to see what she had.

She had given birth to a four-legged set of ears! It was a little female mule. She didn't stand over two feet at the withers, but her ears were at least ten inches long. She was adorable!

Obviously the daughter of a Queen is a Princess, and that's what Vickie called her. That's been several years ago now, and the Balls still own both mother and daughter. Tom has been offered as much as $750 for Princess, a nice return on the $130 he paid for Queenie, but she isn't for sale.

Princess was my first experience with a mule, and it proved to be much more pleasant than the next couple of contacts I had with them. And both were with Tom.

A few years after Princess was born, he came up with a couple of honest-to-goodness, full-sized old plow mules, just like the ones you see on prints at the framing gallery or in the "country-cookin'" restaurants. He picked them up somewhere in the mountains of eastern Kentucky from an old farmer who had finally retired. I wouldn't have believed there were still any plow mules being used in the late 1970s; maybe these were the last two. They were well over sixteen hands and must have weighed at least 1,400 pounds each—very imposing indeed.

He called me out. "Doc, we need Coggins on these two, but one of 'em's got a problem." He showed me a swelling about the size of a baseball on the belly of one, five or six inches behind the left elbow. There was a hairless spot as big as a quarter on the surface of it.

"That looks like an abscess," I said, and reached out toward it. I was standing by the mule's shoulder, facing his rear end. I bent over to get a better look and touched it with my left hand.

The next thing I knew I was flat on my back, seeing stars. Mules, it seems, can cow kick. I vaguely remember being told this by someone now, but I sure didn't remember it then.

I guess if I'd been standing any closer to the mule's rear I wouldn't be writing this today. I'd most likely be arguing my merits with St. Peter just outside the Pearly Gates.

The foot got me in the forehead, just at the forward end of its reach. My forehead swelled to the size of an embedded softball and my whole face turned, over the next few days, first black, then purple and blue, followed by a sickly yellow with a pale greenish tinge. The real fun part, though, came when the swelling gravitated downward to my eyelids, making each one weigh about eight pounds. I had a greatly reduced perspective for several days.

But back to the problem at hand, or at foot. After several minutes I regrouped and began to consider anew the problem of this beast's apparent abscess. I was now sure that's what it was, because it had pretty obviously caused him pain when I touched it. I hadn't really handled it long enough to tell, but I would continue on the assumption that that was what we were dealing with.

So the next step was to lance it to allow drainage. One of the inherent aspects of lancing, however, is the fact that it cannot be achieved without coming in contact with the abscess. If my fingers had hurt him enough for him to kick, what would a scalpel blade induce?

"Pick up his right front leg," I told Tom. "Maybe he won't kick then."

He did as I said. The mule wasn't crazy about his leg being lifted, but he allowed it. Very warily and carefully, standing as far back as I could, I slowly reached toward the abscess with a scalpel and blade. My intention was to make a small jab into the hairless area, but the mule was on to me.

He fired! It was so quick he didn't even lose his balance from the other foot being held up. I had my head out of range, but he caught my left forearm, the one that was reaching for the abscess. He got me right above the wrist and I dropped the scalpel. Other than pain and eventual swelling and discoloration, though, no damage was done.

Horses and, I guess, mules respond well to being "tailed"— forcibly holding the tail up over the back. It turns off the kicking mechanism in most, if you have someone strong enough to do it. Or you can tie a rope to the tail and swing the rope over something and pull hard, thereby exerting some upward pressure; the effect is the same. But this also requires a pretty strong person.

So we tried twitching him. I reached in with a broom handle after the twitch was applied—a procedure that took five full minutes— and he fired just as hard as before.

I told Tom to "ear" him—grab an ear and twist it. This hurts, and I don't like to do it, which was just as well because he wouldn't let us do it anyhow.

Next came tranquilization. He accepted the needle surprisingly well, but I might as well have blown in his ear. He did *not* tranquilize.

I was about ready to give up when Tom made a suggestion. "Doc, why not tie your little blade there to the end of that broomstick and see if you can poke him real quick."

It was worth a try, if I could aim that well. I taped the scalpel, with a new blade—the old one had lost considerable sterility when it was kicked out of my hand earlier—and stood as far away as I could from Lightfoot, as we had begun calling him.

I thrust and he parried. He kicked the broomstick away from his side but I held on to it.

"I don't know, Tom," I said. "He's a lot quicker than I am. And less scared."

"I can't sell him with that thing on him."

"It'll burst on its own in time. Just wait it out," I suggested.

"Doc, you know that I depend on quick turnover to make money. I can't keep him around here for long."

I told him we'd try again. I didn't think we'd succeed; the only time I had even *touched* the abscess was on the first attempt, when I got kicked in the head. All these other times I hadn't gotten within six inches of it.

I armed myself again with the broomstick rapier. Lightfoot was already anticipating his response. I lunged. He kicked. I missed my mark—I actually missed the whole animal—and he missed his, too. Possibly anticipating my target, he had kicked farther inward, actually hitting himself on the side of his own belly.

Or, to be more precise, he kicked himself in the abscess. It ruptured. The problem was solved.

Tom sold Lightfoot and his buddy a few days later for twice what he'd given for them.

Tom had one more mule a few years later. This one was small and young and *wild*.

A man drove into Tom's farm one day towing a large cattle trailer.

"Wanna buy a mule?" he asked. "Cheap."

Now "cheap" is a description of how Tom liked to buy things. "How much?" he asked.

"Twenty-five dollars," the stranger replied.

"Done," Tom rejoined, and went to get a shank so he could lead his newly purchased mule off the trailer.

"Just tell me where you want him. I'll put him there," offered the mule seller.

Tom pointed to a small paddock next to his small barn. "I'll keep him there 'til we get his Coggins."

The man backed his trailer up to the gate and opened it, then swung open the rear of the trailer—and out flew this lightning bolt. Tom said he doesn't think the mule's feet hit the ground for the first thirty feet.

He called me the next day. "Doc, we need to draw a Coggins, but I can't get within twenty feet of the thing."

"Tom, I can't bleed him if you can't catch him," I said.

He called back the next day. "My neighbors helped me chase him into the barn. He's in a stall now."

I naively assumed this meant he had been "caught." "Okay," I said, "I'll be by right after lunch."

He was in a stall, all right, but he was far from "caught." Every time someone entered the stall, or even approached the door, the mule went berserk.

"How'd you get him in there?" I asked.

"Me and about six others chased him 'til he ran in the barn, then we closed the doors and chased him 'til he ran in the stall. I haven't been able to lay a hand on him yet, though."

At each end of Tom's barn, in addition to double sliding doors, were aisle-wide gates that swung inward. With this he could close off the ends of the barn and still allow air to flow through.

"Can you get some of those guys back here? We'll need 'em."

He went to the house and called. In about fifteen minutes, three men showed up.

"That's the craziest thing I ever seen!" said a young man in his twenties.

"Yeah. He'd just as soon run over us as around us. He ain't never been touched, I bet," added an older man, who would have passed for the younger man's twin were it not for a receding hairline and deep crow's feet around his eyes. I guessed they were father and son, and ensuing conversation proved that to be so.

"All right, fellas," I began. "Here's what we need to do. It may not work and we don't want anyone to be hurt, especially the vet, so be careful.

"We'll let him out of the stall and run him down here." I pointed to the end of the barn that opened into the paddock. "If he gets out, at least he'll still be inside a fence.

"One of you stay at the gate, and if we can get him up against the wall, push the gate around and pin him there. Which of you is the strongest?"

"That'd be Elbie," Tom said, nodding toward the stocky young man.

"Okay, Elbie, when the gate's swung around on him, you try to tail him up, but keep the gate between you and him."

"You mean tail him up like a cow?" he asked. These were not horsemen.

"Exactly. And don't let go! Then, Tom, you ear him and I'll try to bleed him."

As with so many things in veterinary medicine, this was easier to describe than to accomplish. Elbie's dad manned the gate, and Tom opened the stall door. Out shot the mule, flying around the barn aisle.

After a few minutes he stopped, and we tried to maneuver him to the desired position. However, it was *our* desired position, not his, and we must have tried for fifteen minutes before getting him there.

Dad swung the gate around, and Elbie tried for the tail but missed, and the mule showed us he had a reverse that was almost as fast as his forward.

And he was not stupid. He now knew where we wanted him, so he wouldn't go there. Another twenty minutes passed before we got him in the proper corner, but this time he turned around before Dad could get the gate around.

Twenty more minutes and we got him in there again. This time, both Dad and Elbie were quicker, and we had him!

Tom grabbed an ear, and the mule swung his head and bopped him in the face, bloodying his nose, but he held on. The mule was trying to sit down, but Elbie held fast and Dad and the other fellow, who remained nameless throughout, leaned hard against the gate.

Now I had to reach through the bars of the gate, try to find his jugular vein and withdraw a few cc's of blood.

This is usually done using a vacuum tube and a double-ended needle. One end of the needle goes into the vein, and once there the other end goes through the rubber stopper of the test tube and the vacuum pulls the blood into the tube. This whole system works very well when the patient is cooperative, but a fractious animal can jerk or fling his head and pull the needle from his neck. If he does this and the tube stopper has already been penetrated, the tube fills with air, and of course the vacuum is gone.

Well, our young mule did exactly this. Even eared and tailed, he was far from still. I lucked out and hit the vein on the first try, but he jumped and I lost the vacuum. This happened on the next try, too, so I used a six-cc syringe to withdraw the blood, which took three tries, and then injected the blood into the tube.

We turned him loose and let him go out in the paddock.

"Doc, how will I ever get him to the stockyards?" Tom asked.

I gave him some tranquilizer granules to put in the mule's feed. These work sometimes and sometimes they don't, but it was worth a try.

I got ready to leave. Tom reached for his wallet.

"How much for that tranquilizer stuff?"

"Eight dollars."

"Okay, so fifteen for the Coggins plus eight; I owe you twenty-three dollars." He counted it out.

I'd been there two hours and had made twenty-three dollars, less expenses.

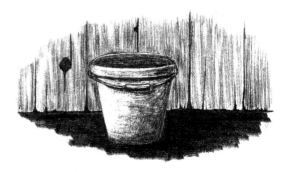

There's an epilogue to this tale. The tranquilizer granules worked, and although the mule did not become a lap dog, Tom and his friends were able to chase him into Tom's trailer a few days later. He was hauled to the stockyards, where Tom continued to feed him the granules. He brought $140.

The little guy was just wild and scared, not mean, and the buyer, a man Tom knew, tamed him and broke him, had him gelded, and took him on trail rides.

It turned out to be a happy ending for everyone.

Tom Ball is still dealing in horses. Princess is still around but getting a little age on her, and she is the only mule I have had any contact with for years. Tom, too, and he says he really doesn't want to see any more.

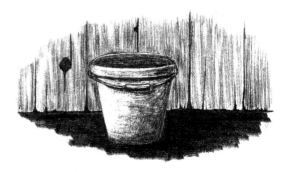

Part Two

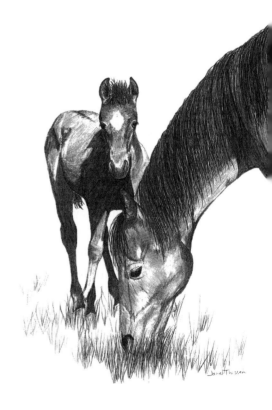

ROBIN, CALICO AND CHICK

This is sort of a flashback.

From the time I was three until I was six, my parents owned a seven-acre "farm," where we kept a couple of horses and various other forms of animal life.

A dog was always present, and at the time we are discussing the resident canine was a black Cocker Spaniel named Robin. There were at least three cats (maybe more; I recall only three). They were all supposed to be barn cats, but I was extremely fond of one, a calico that we had cleverly named Calico. Calico's function as a barn cat was severely compromised by me; I would carry her to the house nearly every day.

One day at the beginning of my six-year-old summer, I was told we were moving. We had sold the seven-acre place and were moving to a ten-acre spread only six miles away. It was even on the same road.

The horses were trailered over. Robin rode over with us in the car.

"When will we bring the cats?" I asked.

"They're not coming," my mother said.

"But they're our cats," I protested.

"We'll get new cats."

"But who will take care of them?"

"We told the people who bought the place that they were there. They were glad to hear it; they said they needed barn cats. They'll take good care of them," Mom explained.

This wasn't particularly well received by me, but six-year-olds rarely have a vote in family matters. I didn't understand this at the time, but since then I have had children of my own, each of whom was six at one time, and now I more fully appreciate my parents' thinking.

The new place had a nicer barn and more paddocks. It also had a creek running through it that abounded in fish (mostly perch and minnows). There were little pools where tadpoles teemed, and it also contained some of nature's most amazing—to a six-year-old—creatures: crawdads.

Overall, this was a good place. But I wanted a cat.

We had been there maybe three weeks and I had asked about acquiring a cat almost daily.

"Wait until we're settled," was the stock answer.

There *was* some confusion, that was sure. A lot of stuff was still in boxes. Looking back now, I see the problem: We'd gone from a house that had a living room, four bedrooms and a den to a house that had a living room, four bedrooms and *no* den. I think the new place was larger, square-foot–wise, but there was a roomful of furniture and other accoutrements that had to be fitted in somewhere.

While in this state of confusion, the farm itself was pretty much ignored. The horses were fed and watered, but that was about it. I was told that the matter of a cat would be attended to in time.

But one morning, after we had been there about three weeks, I got up at my usual time—six or six-thirty—to go outside and play. "Play" consisted of Robin and me going down to the creek to count tadpoles and marvel at crawdads, or just generally to investigate. No one else was ever up when we set off on our treks.

This particular morning, as I stepped out the back door of the kitchen, a cat ran up to me, meowing frantically. It was Calico!

Over the centuries many stories have been written and told about animals that were lost or left behind and that traversed vast distances and finally were reunited with their loved ones. At the age of six I hadn't heard any of them, but since then I believe them all. Calico had only come six miles, and I assume it had taken her three weeks to do it (of course, she may have only started out the night before, for all I knew), but she did it.

I immediately took her in to see my parents and my big brother, all of whom were thrilled to see her at six-thirty in the morning. My brother, who probably wouldn't have gotten up until noon otherwise, was especially overjoyed.

"*Mom!* Get this brat outta here before I break his neck!" I think is how he expressed his delight.

Calico settled in. She joined Robin and me on our expeditions.

There was a very shallow area in the creek where I could walk across and not even get the tops of my feet wet. Robin, of course, splashed through with glee, but the first time Calico went there with us she stayed back, not caring to risk the dangers of the water. She sat there waiting, and when we returned she continued on our rounds with us.

The next time we ventured across the creek, which was probably the next morning, Calico sat quietly until Robin and I had gotten to the other side. I looked back and said, "We'll be back, Calico. Stay there." At which point she leaped into the shallow water!

She got her feet under her, then picked a front paw out of the water and shook it. She put it back down, picked up the other one and shook it, too, then repeated the action with each hind foot. Then she leaped another foot or two and repeated the paw shaking. The creek was probably only six feet wide at this point, so in a couple more bounds she was out on the other side with us. After each forward move, though, she would pick up her paws, one at a time, shake them, then put them back down in the water.

After we finished whatever it is little boys and animals do, we crossed back over the creek, Calico returning in the same manner. But in time she learned that if she walked gingerly instead of leaping, she would splash less, thereby not completely soaking herself. She always shook her paws off after each step, though.

Later that summer there was a fair in the area. I don't know if it was state or county or something totally different, but we all went. It was necessary for me to play all the games they offered, of course; I believe they each cost a dime then. I never won anything; my brother told me no one ever did, and he knew everything. After all, he was fourteen and had been around.

One of the games consisted of what appeared to be a jillion soft drink bottles all pushed up next to each other. For ten cents, participants got to toss three Ping-Pong balls, and if one—only one!—landed atop a bottle, the tosser was a winner.

I watched several people try. My brother and his friend Sonny both tried. The balls bounced on and across the bottles, never even trying to stop. I told Mom I wanted to try. She gave me a dime.

First toss: I missed the bottles entirely. My Ping-Pong ball went straight to the ground.

Second toss: It bounced on and over, the same as the others I had seen.

Third toss: Miracles do still occur! Or at least they did back then. The ball bounced up and around and back and forth and finally came to rest atop a bottle! I won!

Then came the question of what I had won.

The prize turned out to be a baby chick! What a neat prize!

"It'll die," my brother proclaimed.

"Hush, Alan," our mother said. "Honey, you don't really want a chicken, do you?"

"Yes!"

"It'll die," the voice of doom persisted.

"You're just jealous!" I informed him.

We took the chick, which I had named Chick, home and made him a residence in a box in the garage. We placed some water in a mayonnaise jar lid, and my brother got a handful of horse feed, crushed it with a hammer and tossed it in the box with Chick.

Despite the fatal prophecy, Chick lived and thrived and grew—if horses grew as rapidly, they could race as weanlings—and eventually he turned into a rooster. I imagine he had been a rooster all along, but the discovery was exciting nonetheless.

Robin and Calico had discovered Chick early. They showed only mild interest, so when Chick attained the size—and bowel habits—too big for the garage, we had only minimal fear of turning him out in the world.

We carried him outside and put him down in the middle of the backyard. Robin and Calico eyed him with interest but took no action.

We left him out for three or four hours that first day, then put him back in the garage for the night. The next day he would be put out early and left, I was informed.

So the next morning I took him back outside.

Robin and Calico and I left him in the yard and made our rounds. When we returned, Robin spotted Chick from about sixty or seventy feet away and took off toward him, barking ferociously!

Chick, seeing and hearing what must have appeared to be the Hound of Hell, took off as fast as he could, flapping and squawking and making general frantic chicken sounds.

Calico, aware that something was afoot, took off, too, yowling and hissing.

I panicked! I ran toward the house, crying and screaming. Robin was gaining rapidly on Chick, and Calico was right behind him.

Before I could get to the house to rouse some help, Robin caught Chick, jumped on him, and Calico joined in!

There were cat howls and dog growls and chicken squawks. Fur and feathers were flying. And I was sobbing and screaming for them to stop.

And then they did. All three lay there for a moment, panting, and then got up and shook themselves off. I ran over to them and rolled them over and examined them, but, except for a small patch of hair and a feather or two, nobody was hurt.

After a few minutes, Chick got up and crowed and flapped his wings and started running. Calico leaped to her feet instantly. She was after him! Robin began barking and took off, too.

So here's the picture: a rooster running full speed, flapping his wings and making wild chicken sounds, followed by a cat, also at top speed, yowling, followed by a dog, going full out and barking maniacally.

Calico caught Chick just as Robin caught them both. Again, fur and feathers flew from the cloud of dust and din.

And, again, it all stopped and all three combatants lay there gasping. And, again also, all three were unharmed.

They took considerably longer to regroup this time. I went to the house to get Mom, who would probably be up by now. It was after seven.

"Mom, come and see!" I yelled to her.

She came out to the yard just as Chick got up and crowed and flapped. Then he took off, and the whole frantic scene was repeated.

Mom took off after them as I tried to stop her. A six-year-old is no match for a relatively fit thirty-six-year-old, however, and she soon outdistanced me, shouting for Robin to stop, which he did, just as soon as all three crashed into a snarling, growling, squawking heap.

This went on all day. They must have done it fifteen times, and none of them was ever hurt.

That evening I wanted to bring Chick into the garage but was voted down. Mom told Alan to help me take him to the barn. We left him there in a stall with a handful of horse feed.

The next morning I went out to explore with my friends, but Robin and Calico weren't there to greet me. I called for them, and Robin came out of his doghouse and came running to me. And coming out of the doghouse, right behind him, were Calico and Chick.

We investigated about an acre of woods next to the house that morning—and Chick came with us.

As we came back into the back yard, Chick began flapping and crowing and the chase was on again!

This continued several times every day from then on, and each night the unlikely trio would sleep together in Robin's doghouse.

I had always liked animals, but I loved these three. And I think this is when the idea of becoming a veterinarian first entered my mind.

BEDSIDE MANNER

Bedside manner is important in any branch of medicine. It comes naturally to some, but others must learn it. And some never do.

An M.D. doesn't walk up to a patient in a hospital bed and say, "Holy cow! You're sick! You'll never make it!" At least, not many of them do.

That's where the term "bedside manner" came from, of course, but it applies equally to all medical disciplines. A dentist can't say, "Look at those disgusting, rotten teeth! Don't breathe on me! Boy, are you gross!" Well, in truth he can, but he would be wiser taking a softer approach.

Likewise, a veterinarian can't say to a little old lady who has just presented her sixteen-year-old lap dog to him, "Looks like the little cur's about had it. Here's a plastic bag."

Bedside manner did not come naturally to me. I didn't mean to be unkind, and it helped me to know that others had the same problem.

A young man named Art Faries was a senior vet student at my alma mater, and he thought he wanted to go into equine practice. John Emery, in at least his second century on the faculty there, suggested he talk to me.

I was not looking for an associate, nor did I want one. The main reason for this was the workload. Sure, during the breeding season there was enough work to keep two vets busy, but that was only mid-February through the end of June. The other seven-plus months of the year there wasn't enough to keep one man out of trouble.

(The way my practice is set up—as some kind of corporation—I am required to pay unemployment. I am the only employee; I have threatened to lay myself off some July and see if I can collect. Then in January I would rehire myself.)

I told Art Faries that I was not even remotely considering hiring anyone, but then he asked if he could come and make my rounds with me during spring break. That was in March, and March was always pretty busy, so I said he could. We had an extra bedroom, and I could probably introduce him to some of the other horse vets in the area. Maybe he could find a job that way.

He flew in on a Friday evening. He was out for spring break the whole week, so he would be with me for eight full days before he had to fly back the following Sunday.

He was a pleasant young man of around twenty-five, and certainly better prepared to meet the real world than I remembered being at that point. March is still pretty early in the breeding season, but even then the average work day is twelve hours (in April and May it's sixteen). And the work is pretty routine: palping, specking and culturing mares on farm after farm all day long. After a couple of days of this, he commented on the sameness of everything. I told him that's the way of the real world.

At some farms where I thought management and/or ownership would permit, I let him work on a few mares. I would check his palpation evaluations, and most of the time he was pretty accurate in his assessments. He was sharp.

On Wednesday he asked me again, "Is this it? Is this all you ever do?"

"No," I told him, "I worm and vaccinate and treat the occasional colic and suture the occasional laceration, but the reason people call me is to aid in getting their mares in foal, and there's nothing exciting about it."

He sat quietly and appeared to be thinking.

Then the mobile phone made its noise indicating a call. I answered it. When the conversation was over, I told Art, "Now we'll see something a little different."

"What?"

"I'm not sure. That was Joanie McAdams. Remember—we went to her place on Sunday. Her old gelding is acting funny, she said. Maybe he's colicking."

Joanie was an attractive woman in her mid-thirties who trained a few horses in the mornings and tried to run a breeding operation in the afternoons. She had two mares of her own and boarded two for the man whose horses she trained. She also had a pony teaser and Audley, an aged gray gelding that was the first horse she'd ever trained. He was just a pet now, being too old to use for anything else. He was treated better than all the other horses on the place, though, because he was well loved.

We went straight to her farm. Joanie said Audley was "standing funny," which could mean almost anything.

Audley was in his usual paddock, which he shared with the teaser, next to the barn. Joanie met us there.

"He just stands there not moving, all stretched out, like," she said. "He doesn't move or anything. I don't think it's colic."

One look pretty much told the story: sawhorse stance, retracted lips, erect ears, flared nostrils, prolapsed "third eyelid." It was a classic case of tetanus, and a rather advanced one, at that.

"What is it, Grant?" Joanie asked. "Why doesn't he move?"

I was trying to think of some way to break it to her gently. This old horse was very important to her, and he probably wasn't going to make it.

But then Art, wide-eyed, exclaimed, "It's tetanus! It's classic, textbook tetanus! I've never seen a real case! He's going to die!"

Déjà vu.

There was an immediate flashback to many years before, to a time when I was only slightly farther along than Art was now.

I had been out of school and employed as a veterinarian for only a matter of a few weeks when a friend—an architect—was passing through the area on his way home from a business trip. He called me.

"Grant, this is Ned. I'm in Alexandria, and I thought I'd take an extra day and come visit."

This was great. He had gotten through school a few years before me (he didn't have the inconvenience of four years of vet school) and moved off to the big city to make his fortune. We didn't see each other very often, and I really liked Ned. I gave him directions on how to find me.

He spent the night, and the next day he said he'd like to ride with me as I made my rounds. It was a relatively light and routine schedule: I had only six calls on the book.

We headed out, and everything went smoothly—encephalitis vaccinations for a band of eight horses, worming three at another farm, castrating a calf, TB testing for about a dozen head of cattle and so on. Really ordinary stuff.

Late in the morning I got a call on the mobile radio. "Base to unit two. Grant, go to Lucy Kidwell's place. She's got a horse acting funny and she needs someone to look at it."

I didn't know Lucy Kidwell. I didn't know 75 percent of the practice's clientele at this point. Richard, my employer, had told everyone about me and introduced me to a few, but basically I was given directions to each place and presented myself as Dr. Spencer's associate when I got there.

I talked back to the radio. "Edna, where is Lucy Kidwell? And is it an emergency?"

"She says she'd like someone right away," Edna responded, and then gave me directions.

I was still learning my way around the county, so it took me longer than it should have to get there. When we did arrive, I introduced myself to a plain young woman—maybe late twenties, but I'm terrible at ages—who was obviously distressed at the length of time it had taken me to get there.

She took me to a nondescript, medium-size gelding and said, "He's not moving right." She led him a few steps.

He wasn't moving right, and there were considerable other abnormalities as well. In fact, he was almost a textbook case, not quite as obvious as Audley, but pretty close.

"This horse has rather advanced tetanus," I proclaimed. "He's gonna die."

I thought Lucy was going to keel over. Her eyes filled with tears.

"Get out of here!" she shouted. "Get off my farm!"

I had no idea what her problem was. As I got back in the car, I said, "His only chance is to put him in a dark stall and give him high levels of penicillin."

"Get out of here!" she screamed, and burst into tears.

As we drove away, Ned said, "Maybe you should have handled that differently."

That was pretty obvious, I thought, but it still hadn't occurred to me what I had done wrong. I said as much.

"Bedside manner, dummy," he explained. "You can't just walk up to a person you've just met and tell her that her horse is gonna die."

"But it is," I protested.

"But you can't just blurt it out. You have to soften it."

Later that day I stopped by the office (Richard's house). Richard was there.

"Grant, Lucy Kidwell called. I just got back from there," he told me.

"Her horse has tetanus."

"Yes. And he's probably going to die. We've started him on penicillin and he's in a boarded-up stall, but I don't think it'll do any good.

"A couple of months ago," he continued, "her father died of a heart attack. Her mother's been diagnosed as having terminal cancer. The day before you came here, her dog was run over and killed.

"Now, two minutes after you meet her, you tell her that her horse—her *favorite* horse—is going to die." I'm sure he was angry, possibly irate, but he was talking to me as calmly as if he was just giving me directions to another farm. "Grant, even if she'd just been named Queen of the May, you can't do that."

I never did it again.

≋

But back to the present. Joanie stared open-mouthed at Art for a moment, then said, matter-of-factly, "He is not going to die." Tears came to her eyes.

"Joanie," I said, "he's right. Audley has tetanus. There's very little chance from what we see here, but we'll do all we can." I gave Art a dirty look.

"He *will* die," Art insisted. "Just look at him. There's no chance!"

Joanie's tears began flowing. Art looked puzzled. "What's wrong?" he asked.

We treated Audley. We placed him in a dark stall, gave him a high dose of tetanus antitoxin and began him on high levels of penicillin, but it was too late. He couldn't swallow (remember, tetanus is lockjaw), and in a couple of days Joanie chose to have him put to sleep rather than see him starve. It was the right choice. She said she didn't want Art to be there when we performed the euthanasia.

I explained bedside manner to Art. I probably wasn't as angry with him as Richard must have been with me, and he said, yes, he could see where maybe he shouldn't say it quite so bluntly. "But I was right!" he insisted. "I don't see why she was so upset."

As I said, Art was sharp. He went back to school the next Sunday (the day after I put Audley down) and eventually graduated third in his class (I didn't have that problem). Instead of entering the boring real world, though, he received an internship at another university and decided to stay in academia. Bedside manner is not nearly as important there.

THE MARE

My mobile phone made its sound signifying an incoming call. It was something between a ring and a buzz. I answered.

"Doc, this is Walt Reynolds. I wanted you to hear this from me before you heard it from somebody else. We couldn't breed that mare. She was crazy. I've never seen anything like it."

I'd sent a few mares to be bred over the years that had acted up. Sometimes they were nervous or frightened or, occasionally, just plain mean, but I'd never been called about it before. She must have really put on a show.

Walt was the manager of Greenhills Farm, which stood possibly the finest group of stallions ever assembled in one place at one time.

"That mare" was Masonica, a four-year-old owned by Stanislas Craft of New York. Stan was in his seventies or eighties and had been in the horse business for close to half a century. He had bred twenty-five or thirty stakes winners, and Masonica was one of them. She'd won a small stakes race at two and nearly $100,000 and was possibly the weak link in her pedigree. Her dam had produced five stakes winners.

Stan had cut back on his broodmares. He now owned six, and the ones he bred in Kentucky he sent to me during the breeding season. He was a great boarder; he had an idea in his head of how much it should cost to board a mare and his idea was four dollars a day more than I normally charged, so he insisted on paying me his figure instead of mine.

This particular year I had five of his mares (one had been sent to Florida): four foaling mares and Masonica, who was only about three months off the racetrack. She had chipped a bone in an ankle and he'd decided against surgery.

Stan bred to the best stallions. Masonica was to be bred to Dragon's Lair, who was in his first year of stud duty. He had only raced a few times, then retired undefeated after an injury in training. His stud fee was in the range of $50,000, and his book was full, with a waiting list.

I thanked Walt for calling and apologized for the problem, but I didn't understand it.

Masonica and the other mares had arrived at my farm about two weeks earlier, in late February. We had given her a couple of days to get used to the new routine and then began teasing her.

"Teasing" is a procedure done to see if a mare is receptive to a stallion. Every farm has a "teaser," a gentle stallion that is led to the mares so they can see, hear and smell him.

Normally a mare will not want to have a stallion around. She'll pin her ears or run at him or kick at him, but if she is "in season"— that is, in the time of her cycle when she is willing to be bred—she will stand quietly or even back up to the stallion with her tail raised and will squat and urinate.

After about a week, Masonica began showing to Patches, our teaser. She didn't show real well, but there was no question that she was in season. Patches loved her, and I never recall him being fooled.

By performing certain examinations on her, I determined the correct time for breeding her would be in two days, and then I called Greenhills to arrange an appointment (called "booking" because it's written down in a book) for the correct day.

The next morning we jumped her. This is pretty much as it sounds: We restrained her and allowed Patches to mount her. Many a maiden (a mare that has never been bred) thinks little of this procedure, but Masonica didn't seem to mind. She wiggled a little but put up no real resistance.

The next morning we jumped her again and I examined her once more before she went off to be bred. Everything was great; all we had to do was get her to Dragon's Lair and she would be in foal. Or so I thought.

The van picked her up at quarter to eight, and Laurie, the girl who worked for me, went with her as she did with all the mares when they were bred.

Walt's call came about nine-fifteen, and evidently things had not gone well.

A few minutes later, around nine-twenty-five, the phone made its alien sound again. It was Laurie.

"Grant, they couldn't breed Masonica. She was terrible! I never saw anything like it!"

It sounded a great deal like what Walt had said. I told her I'd be home in an hour or so and we'd check her.

Most mares gradually stop being receptive to a stallion after they ovulate, but occasionally one reacts as if someone had flipped a switch. When ovulation occurs, these will no longer stand to be bred. Maybe Masonica was one of these.

I got home around eleven. Laurie told me the Greenhills office had called and said we could bring Masonica back tomorrow if she was still in season, but if we did they wanted me to come with her.

I examined her. I was sure there was no way she would still be breedable tomorrow.

I told Laurie we'd jump her again. Laurie was a good worker and loved horses and was game for almost anything.

"Grant," she said, "you didn't see her at the breeding shed. She was crazy!"

I told her she could handle Patches and I'd handle Masonica. She agreed, but reluctantly.

Masonica didn't bat an eye. She didn't even shift weight.

"Laurie, what went on there?" I asked.

"Just the normal stuff. She was fine until they brought the stud in, and then she went crazy. People were running everywhere. She got away from them and started chasing everything."

Got away from them? The best-run, most experienced breeding shed crew in all of Kentucky? Wow.

Sure enough, when I checked her the next morning it was too late to breed her. I called the Greenhills office and told Sondra we wouldn't be there. Sondra was the woman who handled the bookings, and she was far and away the nicest, most cordial, most helpful booking person in the area.

She said, "Dr. Kendall, Walt has asked, when she does return—whenever it is—that you come with her. I didn't see it, but everyone told me they'd never seen anything like it."

I assured her that I'd be there, whenever it was. This was something I had to see.

There is a hormone injection that can be given to bring a mare back in season sooner than she would normally return if left on her own. I decided not to give one to Masonica. Stan didn't care if his mares foaled very early, and I really don't like January or February foalings. It's just too cold most of the years, and it's rough on the newborn. It's also rough on the guy attending the mare, and as this would most likely be me, I just let her come back in season on her own. (However, although I don't *like* early foals, I won't refuse to breed a mare that comes into a nice, normal heat period early in the season—which is what I thought Masonica had done.)

Sixteen days after she had gone out of season, Masonica again became interested in Patches and he in her. Examination revealed everything to be normal again. The exam indicated that she should be bred in two more days, so I called Greenhills to book her to Dragon's Lair for the correct day.

"Hi, Sondra. This is Grant Kendall. I need to book a mare."

"Is this *THE* mare, Dr. Kendall?" she asked.

"I'm afraid so. Can we breed her the day after tomorrow?"

"Yes. She's on the book. Remember, you need to accompany her."

"Thanks. We'll all be there."

The next day we jumped her again, but Laurie still wouldn't hold her. Examination on the morning of her scheduled breeding showed everything to be in great shape.

The van arrived right on time to pick her up for the trip to Greenhills. Jack, one of the regular drivers for the commercial van service that we used, had not been the driver when Masonica went before. "Is this *THE* mare?" he asked as we loaded her. "They tell me she was really something."

I saw Laurie and Masonica off and drove over to Greenhills in my car. I parked by the farm office so I wouldn't be in the way of the vans. Greenhills stood about two dozen very popular stallions, and it was likely there would be at least twenty vans in there over the next half hour.

I got out of my car and started walking up toward the stallion barn. Laurie had unloaded Masonica and was a few yards ahead of me.

A car pulled up behind me and stopped. "Hey, Grant!" a voice called.

I turned around. It was Rick Edwards, Greenhills' resident vet and a good friend. "Is that *THE* mare?" he continued, pointing to Masonica.

I told him that she was.

"Boy," he said, "I want to see this! I was taking care of a sick foal last time and missed it. They tell me they'd never seen anything like it."

"That's what I hear, Rick. I have a syringe full of tranquilizer in my pocket, just in case."

Walt Reynolds walked down from the breeding shed. "Doc Kendall, I need to ask you to let us breed this gal last. We need to get the rest of 'em bred before we get somebody killed." Then he added, "I've never seen *anything* like that before."

I told Laurie to take Masonica out of line and be patient. We had been the third ones there, so it would be a while.

A few minutes later, another van arrived. The driver, a young man named Ronnie, had hauled for me from time to time. He hopped out of the cab and shouted, "Hey, Doc! Is that *THE* mare?"

And after another few minutes, a fellow I had never seen before brought a mare in. As he walked by, he nodded toward Masonica. "Is that *THE* mare?" he asked. Her fame had spread.

As the other mares were bred—there were twenty-one of them that morning—I noticed an unusually large number of Greenhills uniforms standing around. I commented on it to Rick.

"It looks like the word's gotten out," he said. "Everyone wants to see the show. I bet half the farm's employees are here."

Finally, the last mare before us was bred. Walt called us to come up to the small holding barn where they kept a teaser. Laurie was obviously getting very nervous, so I took Masonica and put her in the stall that Walt had indicated.

They slid open a window between her stall and the adjacent one, where their teaser was. Everything went fine. The teaser made some sexy comments in horse talk and the mare said something like "Your place or mine," also in horse.

"This went fine the last time, too," said Walt, then asked me to bring her out so they could jump her. He brought out the teaser and, again, all went well. Greenhills had a policy of jumping all incoming maidens; they had done this the last time, also. "So far, so good," Walt said.

There was a crowd of several dozen people up near the breeding shed. Most were Greenhills employees, but there were several who had been there to breed. They had put their mares back in the vans and were staying for the fireworks. Sondra, from the Greenhills office, was also there.

I led Masonica up the path to the shed. As we walked through the big double doors, the entire breeding shed crew took a collective step backward. "That's *THE* mare," someone whispered.

Walt spoke. "We're gonna try this mare with a minimum of bodies here. She needs all the room she can get." Then he named three or four of the crew and told them to step outside. They smiled as they left.

The young man who handled the mares for breeding took Masonica from me very carefully and placed her in a stanchion, where she was washed and her tail was wrapped. He brought her out, and they twitched her and put on a leg strap. These are routine precautions taken at the time of breeding because stallions are often worth millions of dollars and if the mare kicks she could injure him or one of the men working with the horses. From what I had been told, these restraints had not stopped Masonica the last time.

Everyone was moving very cautiously and deliberately. A muscle twitch or a flick of her tail caused everyone to jump.

You could see the tension in all the faces.

While all this was going on, the stud man had gone to get Dragon's Lair from his stall in the adjacent stallion barn. He walked him up to the double doors of the breeding shed and stopped. Or, I should say, the horse stopped! I don't know if it was the sight or the scent, but as soon as Dragon's Lair became aware of Masonica, he refused to move forward.

"She darn near cleaned his clock last time," murmured Walt nervously. "I imagine he remembers."

The stallion wouldn't enter the breeding shed. After considerable pulling and rear slapping, they turned him around and tried to back him in. That didn't work, either. They blindfolded him to no avail—he wasn't going to enter that building!

Finally they took the twitch and strap off Masonica. Carefully. She just stood there.

Walt told two of the men to cradle the stallion in. The two men locked arms behind the horse, and with the stud man pulling on the shank, they manhandled him through the doorway.

The twitch and strap were again carefully applied to Masonica. With much shoving and pulling, Dragon's Lair was maneuvered over to her.

"This is where it all broke loose," Walt whispered, "as soon as he touched her."

You could almost taste the tension in the air.

Dragon's Lair sniffed her. She raised her tail, and everyone within ten yards jumped back. But she just stood there; he hadn't touched her yet.

The crew prepared the stallion for breeding. It appeared to be a much quicker wash than usual, and the guy doing it kept glancing over his shoulder at Masonica.

They manipulated Dragon's Lair back toward her. He sniffed her again. He liked what he smelled.

"Be careful, boys," Walt warned. "We don't want anybody hurt."

Still, Dragon's Lair had not touched her. But then, all of a sudden, he reared, lunged forward and bred her. She didn't bat an eye.

"I'll be a son of a gun," said Walt.

The following March, Masonica had a beautiful chestnut filly.

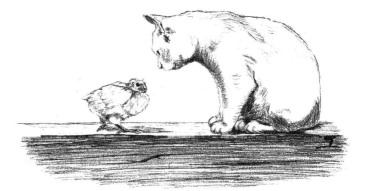

IGNORANCE

"Ignorance is bliss."

I don't know who said that, nor do I know if it's really true. If it is, however, I've had some ecstatically happy clients.

Frequently, ignorance is not harmful; it may even be a little bit funny.

One of the things that separates the human race from other species is the timing of mating. In the so-called lower forms of animal life, mating is done only when the female is receptive, and this receptiveness is timed so that the ensuing offspring will arrive at a time when its survival can be somewhat assured.

For instance, in the natural state, horses, with a gestation of around eleven months, mate in June, July and August. The young, therefore, arrive in May, June and July, when the weather is warm and the grass is growing and there is plenty of it to eat.

Large cats (lions, tigers, etc.), on the other hand, have a gestation of about three and a half months. Consequently, they mate in February and March so their young will also arrive around May or June, when the weather is warm and the grass is growing and there are plenty of baby horses to eat. (It's a jungle out there.)

People, however, will mate at any time of the year, with no thought as to what will be going on in the world nine months later when it comes time to bring forth the result of said mating. In fact, it's been shown that the onset of the TV rerun season in February and March usually results in a high number of births in November and December, hardly an optimum time to ensure survival if the births occurred in the wild. (However, if humans lived in the wild, it's unlikely TV reruns would be much of a factor.)

Floyd Yokum was a postal worker who had a filly he trained and tried to race. She couldn't outrun you or me, and her racing career was one of little distinction (she never won a race), so Floyd decided to do what countless others before him had done: breed her. This, in itself, is pretty ignorant: Why would a person want to reproduce a failure? I mean, Mr. Ford did not come out with Edsel, Mark II. There has been no multimillion-dollar production of *Son of Ishtar*. However, this is the nature of horse people: If she can't run, breed her.

This really isn't something I should complain about. My main function in life is to assist people in getting their mares to reproduce. If only those mares that actually *should* be bred *were* bred, I might well be unemployed, as the number of broodmares would probably decrease by 65 or 70 percent.

This desire to breed his mare is not where Floyd showed ignorance, though. This is probably no more than a combination of misguided judgment and the hope we all have for the future. Floyd's ignorance lay in how he approached this proposed mating.

One spring day I was at the local Thoroughbred training center where Floyd had his filly. Her name was Dora's Darling (Dora was Floyd's wife). I was getting some medication out of my car for a horse with a respiratory condition when Floyd approached me.

"Doc," he said, "I think I'm gonna breed Dora."

Although I couldn't be sure, I felt certain he meant the filly, and wasn't telling me his plans for that evening at home. Not knowing exactly the response he expected, I said simply, "Okay."

"What do I need to do?" he asked.

Now I knew he meant the mare. Floyd and Dora had two children.

"Well, you need to choose a stallion and get a contract," I told him.

"I did that. I got a contract for Gametime." He beamed. Gametime was one of those stallions whose popularity for breeding seemed to be maintained for no apparent reason, because his foals neither sold nor raced well.

"Okay," I said. "Now you have to determine the time to breed her to him."

"I'm off tomorrow. Can I breed her then?"

"Gee, Floyd, I don't know. Is she in?" When talking to a horse breeder, "in" means "in heat"—in other words, receptive to the stallion. To a racetracker, though, it means is she "in" a race.

"No," he replied. "I'm not gonna run her anymore, so can I breed her tomorrow?"

I was beginning to have concerns about this conversation. "I mean, is she in heat?" I asked. "Have you teased her?"

Straightfaced, he answered, "Doc, you know I don't mistreat her, and as far as heat, heck, it's only about sixty degrees. Does it have to be hot?"

It took me a second to grasp what he meant about not mistreating her, but I saw immediately that he knew nothing about breeding cycles. I even wondered a moment exactly how he and Dora had had those two kids. I began to explain the birds and bees as they pertain to horses.

"A mare is only breedable for a few days every few weeks, Floyd. They have what is called an estrous cycle, and it lasts about three weeks. The time to breed her is at the point when she likes the stallion the most. That point is called being in heat."

He interrupted me. "She's never seen Gametime. She doesn't know if she likes him or not. Should I take her to him?"

I was beginning to understand why mail delivery was so slow and erratic.

"No, Floyd. She'll like him if she's in heat. You need to start teasing her." He began to interrupt again, undoubtedly to tell me he doesn't mistreat her, but I put my hand up to quiet him and continued. "'Teasing' is when you bring a stallion to her and watch her reaction. If she tries to bite or kick, she's not in heat, but if she raises her tail and turns around and presents her rear end to him, then she *is* in heat. And that's when you want to breed her."

"You mean I have to bring Gametime here? Will they let me do that?"

I looked Floyd up and down, trying to find the hidden microphone, then glanced around to see if I could find where the Candid Camera was hidden. This couldn't be real. But then I looked Floyd in the eyes; he was serious.

"No, you can use any stallion." He started to say something, and I knew it was about having a contract to Gametime and not wanting another stallion, so I continued quickly. "The stallion is just to see if she's in heat; you'll still breed her to Gametime."

"Where do I find a stallion?"

"Floyd, for goodness' sake! This is a training center! There are more than a thousand horses here! Ask some of the trainers if someone has something you can tease with." Teasing with a horse in training is not a really good idea, but it's done often with no ill effects.

"Okay. I'll find one. After I tease her, can I breed her tomorrow? I'm off work then."

This conversation continued for quite a while longer, but we can leave it here. This example of ignorance was pretty funny (to me) and no one was hurt, but all too often ignorance brings harm, and it's usually to an animal.

(I'm sure you're dying to know: Dora's Darling was not bred "tomorrow" but eventually did get in foal to Gametime and produced a filly named Darling Dora, which raced almost as well and successfully as her dam. After two years of trying to win a race with her— and failing—Floyd made a broodmare out of her, too.)

The first case of pure ignorance I saw occurred only a few weeks after I left school. As related earlier, at this time I was employed by a large-animal practice in beautiful northern Virginia. Although my employer let me do most of the horse work in the practice, there were still cows that needed my attention. I've gone on record as saying I don't like cattle, but not liking something and wishing it harm are two different things. Cows can rule the world for all I care; just don't expect me to vote for one.

It was a Saturday morning. I had just wormed a half-dozen horses, and I was leaving the small farm when the mobile radio squawked.

"Base to unit two. Base to unit two. Come in, unit two." Richard, my employer, was unit one; "base" was his kitchen, the voice that of Edna, his wife. I never understood why she just couldn't say, "Grant, speak to me," but it was always, "Base to unit two."

"Unit two here," I replied. That's the way I was told to answer. I'd have preferred to say, "Here I am, Edna," but that would have been frowned upon.

"Unit two, go to Wally Pepperdine's place. He thinks a cow is calving."

I didn't know Wally Pepperdine or his place, but Edna told me what road it was on, and I found it. It turned out to be a small farm, maybe ten acres.

Wally Pepperdine, I learned later, was an attorney who worked in Arlington, just outside of Washington, D.C., about a forty-five-minute drive from where he lived. It being a Saturday, he was home, and he greeted me as I pulled up to his barn. He looked like something out of a 1940s English movie: fiftyish, tweed cap, tweed jacket, sweater, wool trousers—a typical British peer surveying his baronial estate. I looked at his clothes and wanted to say, "Man, don't you know it's July?" but I didn't. I did ask the whereabouts of the cow.

He pointed to the side of the barn. There, about a hundred yards from us, was a cow lying flat on her side.

"Are you sure she's calving?" I asked, as I began getting equipment out.

"Pretty sure," he answered. "She's overdue."

"When was she due?"

"At the same time these others were," he said, motioning to five other cows with calves grazing around the barn.

I looked at them. These were good-sized calves. "How old are those?" I asked.

"Oh, let's see. They came in May. About two months, I guess."

"And this cow was due to calve then? Surely not."

"Oh, yes. I don't understand why she's so late."

"How do you know she was due then?"

"The bull was only with them in August and early September. Nine months would have been May."

"Do you know she's pregnant?"

"Yes. They were all checked in October."

"Mr. Pepperdine, a cow *doesn't* carry a calf eleven months."

I had gathered all of what I thought I might need, and headed through the gate and toward the down cow. Pepperdine came as far as the gate. As I got nearer to the cow, I began detecting an odor. When I was within fifty feet of her, it began to be overpowering, and by the time I got to her, I was feeling nauseous.

I have a strong stomach. Sights and smells that have caused people around me to barf have only caused a slight queasiness in me. I did not throw up this time, either, but I have never been as close.

My vocabulary should be sufficient to describe the stench, but it isn't. You wouldn't want to read it anyhow. If you take the worst smell you've ever encountered and multiply it by five, you'll be close. Maybe.

She stank so badly that I was feeling lightheaded. I put my hand on her side, more to steady myself than anything. She was *hot!* I didn't take her temperature, but it must have been astronomical.

I looked at her vulva. Oozing out was a thick, grayish-brown stream of slime, which appeared to be the source of the odor. It was so bad now that my eyes were watering.

I put on a plastic sleeve and inserted my arm into her vagina. About six or eight inches in I felt bone. I grasped it and pulled.

Out came part of a leg. There was no identifiable tissue attached, just gross, slimy putrefaction. I reached back in and removed another leg bone, then a skull, another leg, some vertebrae, a few ribs, another leg. Eventually I had removed an entire calf skeleton, with all the soft tissue decomposed. The procedure took nearly half an hour, and by the time I was finished I had the gross guck all over me. I medicated the cow's uterus and put her on systemic antibiotics.

I told Pepperdine what had happened. "She must have tried to calve weeks ago," I said, "and evidently the calf was malpositioned and couldn't be delivered by her. After a while, the uterine contractions stop and the calf dies and decomposes.

"Didn't she show any signs earlier?"

"Well . . ." He appeared to be thinking. "Yes, maybe. Back when the others were calving, I remember she laid around for a day or two. I did notice she was beginning to smell a little recently."

"Why didn't you call back then?"

"Well, like I said, after a couple days she got up and started eating again. Like everything was all right."

I told him I'd be back Sunday morning to see how she was and to treat her again.

As I drove from Sir Pepperdine's estate, I picked up the mobile radio's microphone.

"Unit two to base. Come in, Edna."

"Base here, unit two. You're supposed to say, 'Come in, base.'"

"Okay. Come in, base."

"Base here."

"Call my next appointment and tell 'em I'll be late. I have to shower and change." I told her why.

Early the next morning, Wally Pepperdine called the office, i.e., Richard's home. The cow had died. He told Richard that she had been fine until I "fooled around" in her and gave her those shots.

It was more than a year later when I came across the next serious case of ignorance. I stopped at a fast-food restaurant for lunch, and as I was carrying my tray and looking for a seat, I heard my name called.

"Doc Kendall," someone said, "join us."

I looked around and saw Lenny Albertson sitting with someone I didn't know. Lenny is one of the world's nice guys. He always smiles, never gets in a hurry, likes everyone, is never bothered by anything. I had been there in Virginia for over a year and had met him shortly after I arrived. He would often ride with me when he had nothing else to do, which was most of the time.

Lenny didn't work, per se; that is to say, he didn't have a job. He would occasionally help one brother on his cattle farm and sometimes he'd help his other brother, who owned a feed store, but mostly Lenny visited and talked. Except on weekends.

On weekends, Lenny played polo. It was his passion. Evidently he was pretty good, too. And he should have been. When that was pretty much all a forty-year-old man had done for twenty years, proficiency sets in.

But this isn't about Lenny. He was not ignorant. In fact, he may be one of the four or five most intelligent, aware people I have ever known.

I sat down with Lenny and the other man.

"Doc, this is Ed," said Lenny. "He's got a problem with a horse."

I offered my hand. "Grant Kendall," I said.

"Ed Brewer. You're a vet?"

"Yeah."

"I've got a yearling that's not doing well," he told me.

Everyone wants free advice. Everywhere I go, and I'm sure everywhere any vet goes, as soon as it's known I'm a vet, people begin asking questions.

"If you're having problems, you should have your vet check him out," I said, trying to avoid the questions I knew were coming.

"I don't have a vet. Lenny said I should talk to one."

Oh me, I thought. "Okay, what's the problem?"

"He's not doing well. He keeps losing weight. What do you think it is?"

"I have no idea. It would be very helpful if I could see him."

"I'll tell you about him. I bought him last year at the sale here." There was a small annual Thoroughbred sale in the area. "I plan to race him, but he has never done well. I feed him a lot of hay, but he doesn't eat it well at all. What can I do?"

"Golly, without seeing the horse and examining him, I can't begin to tell you."

"What'll you charge to see him?"

I explained that there would be a charge for going to his place and then a charge for any diagnostic work and/or treatment that might be necessary.

He thought for a minute, then said, "I think I'll give him a little more hay. If he doesn't pick up in a couple of weeks, maybe I'll call you."

I told him that would be fine and felt certain I'd never hear from him again.

But I was wrong.

Three days later he called. Or, I should say, three *nights* later he called. It was after eleven and I was asleep.

"This is Ed Brewer. My yearling is not doing any better. Can you come see him?"

I told him I'd be by in the morning.

"I won't be here," he said. "I work. Can you come now?"

I explained the time to him and asked him what time he came home from work. Five-thirty. I said I'd see him then and asked where he lived.

At about a quarter of six the next evening I found the address he had given me. I thought I was at the wrong place; this wasn't a farm. It was a small brick house sitting on maybe an acre or so and there was no barn or fencing in sight.

I picked up the mobile mike to call Edna and ask if she could check the address for me, but before I could contact her, Brewer came out of the house.

"He's out back," he said. "You'll have to walk around the house."

I followed him, and when we reached the backyard I saw the yearling.

He was lying on his side in the yard. His head was flat on the ground, but he was moving it around, taking bites of the grass. A few feet behind him was a small pen, maybe fifteen feet square, with the planks broken on the side nearest the colt.

He was a hide-covered skeleton. If you've ever seen pictures in *National Geographic* of animals that died from drought or starvation, you know what he looked like. I was so stunned by what I saw I didn't realize that Brewer was speaking. I asked him to repeat.

"I said, he broke out of his corral last night. That's why I called. He's just laid there ever since, biting at the grass." The colt had eaten the grass down to the dirt as far as he could reach with his mouth, but obviously had not gotten up. There were a few hard, dry fecal balls by his rear and what was apparently a small puddle of urine by his belly.

I looked at the "corral." It was dirt, that part of it which wasn't covered with manure. There was no shelter. A bucket with slimy green water hung from a post. In one corner was a pile of dead grass.

"You kept him in here?" I asked. Brewer nodded. "All the time?" I asked again. Brewer nodded again.

"You bought him at the sale last fall—almost a year ago—and he's been in this little pen ever since?"

"Yes," said Brewer.

"There's no shelter," I pointed out.

"I know. I wanted to make him tough."

"The water's filthy."

"That stuff's good for him. It's got vitamins and minerals."

"It's got bacteria and algae. What's this stuff?" I asked, pointing to the dead grass.

"That's his hay. I give him a lot, but he just doesn't eat much of it. I've got a whole big pile of it over there." He pointed to a decaying mound of dead grass a few yards beyond the pen.

I walked over and picked up a handful. "This isn't hay. This is just dead grass and weeds. How much grain do you give him?"

"I don't give him grain. I give him lots of hay."

I went back to the colt. I bent down by him and listened to his heart through my stethoscope. He made no attempt to move. His heart was beating rapidly but weakly. I pinched the skin on the side of his neck, and the pinch stayed in the skin—a sign of dehydration. He rolled his eye that was off the ground toward me and let out a very feeble nicker.

The colt was starving to death. Or maybe he already had. I could see no way to save him.

I looked around the yard. It was a nice yard, nearly an acre of well-growing grass. I looked again at the filthy sty that was the colt's pen—a small prison within this beautiful lawn. I hadn't noticed before, but all around the outside of the pen the grass had been chewed down to the dirt as the colt had reached under the planks as far as he could in an attempt to get something to eat. Maybe I was anthropomorphizing, but I think he finally broke out in desperation, trying to get something edible.

"What's his problem? Why is he losing weight?" Brewer asked.

I was already very upset, and I was getting very angry. I wanted to lock Brewer in a cage in the middle of a five-star restaurant and feed him nothing but uncooked macaroni for a year. I was so angry that tears were forming.

"He's starving to death," I said.

"No, he's not! I give him lots of hay and he won't even eat it! There's something wrong with him!"

"Yes," I agreed. "He's starving to death."

A deep hollow moan emanated from the colt. I looked down at him. He had stopped biting at the grass. I put my stethoscope over his heart.

It wasn't beating. He was dead.

"You let him die!" yelled Brewer. "You just stood there and let him die!"

About a week later I saw Lenny in his brother's feed store.

"Doc, that fella Brewer's not happy. Says you wouldn't do anything for his colt. Just let him die. Says it'll be a cold day in July when he pays your bill or ever calls another vet."

"I'm sure he's right on both counts, Lenny. And it'll be a hot day in January before I'll go to his place again."

"He says he's gonna try again this fall. Thinks he'll buy a filly this time."

A few weeks later I packed up the family and moved to Kentucky to start my own practice, so I don't know if Brewer bought another horse. I could have found out, but I really didn't want to know. I hope he didn't.

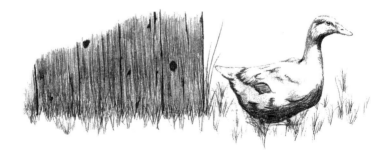

BARNEY

"Doc, I got things to do over at the mare barn. I'll see you there when you're done here." He seemed unusually downcast.

Rufus was the farm manager—a working farm manager. *Nothing*—absolutely nothing—was done to a horse of Woodhill Farm unless Rufus was present. This is the way it had been for the seven or eight years I had been the farm's vet, and I'd been told it had been that way ever since he'd been named manager more than twenty years before.

But here he was, telling me to do what I needed to do here at Barn 3, the small barn that housed the pleasure horses and pensioners, without overseeing it.

He drove off over the hill. I turned to Whitey, Rufus's assistant, and said, "I never thought I'd be able to touch a horse on this farm without Rufe watching me."

"He just ain't got the heart for it, Doc," Whitey replied.

"Heart for what?"

"Mrs. Wharton says to put Barney down."

I couldn't believe it. I asked him to repeat it. I'd heard correctly. "Put Barney down" is what he'd said.

"Are you sure?" I asked.

"Yeah, Doc, I'm afraid so. The old guy's just not getting around like he used to, and he's not seeing too good—he's bumping into trees and stuff."

I walked into the barn and down the aisle to Barney's stall. The old boy was in there peacefully chewing on a little hay. In all the years I'd known him, everything Barney had done had been done peacefully.

Barney was around thirty-two years old, we were pretty sure. Mrs. Wharton, Woodhill's owner, was the only person who could remember a day when Barney wasn't on the farm. Cynthia, Mrs. Wharton's older daughter, was thirty-two, and supposedly the two-year-old Barney was a second-birthday present for Cynthia, a gift from her father. Gerald Wharton had passed away a few years ago.

Barney was a solid, plain brown gelding about the size of a Welsh pony, but a little more refined. The only white was a very small star on his forehead. If nothing else, he was memorable to me as one of the few pony-size equidae that had lived long and remained unfoundered. (One of my teachers in vet school had told me there were two kinds of pony: those that had foundered and those that will. Over the years, these had been words to live by.)

Cynthia had learned to ride on Barney. Claudia, the younger Wharton daughter, had also learned on his gentle, safe back. Both girls went on to bigger, fancier mounts over the years, but Barney's usefulness did not lessen.

He was trained to pull a cart and would appear in the local annual Christmas parade; in fact, he hadn't missed one for almost twenty-five years.

And even though the Wharton girls grew into larger mounts, his use as a riding horse didn't end. Rufe's three kids had all learned their early horsemanship with Barney—as had Whitey's son as well.

Cynthia's two children, now about eight and five, and Claudia's six-year-old had also been introduced to riding by Barney. And a few years ago, when my daughter had shown an interest in having a horse, I took her out to Woodhill several times to ride Barney, to see if the interest was really there. We'd saddle him up—he was probably twenty-three or twenty-four then—and sit her up on him; she was about five. Then we'd turn them loose in a paddock. As long as he felt the weight on his back, Barney would walk, quietly and slowly. If the weight left, as it did when Janie would overadjust as he made a turn, he would stop. She would fall off; he would stop.

But Barney's usefulness was not limited to being ridden and driven by children. He was the best babysitter I've ever seen. You could put him with the wildest weanlings in the world and somehow he'd become their friend and surrogate. To catch even the most contrary babies, all that was necessary was to call Barney.

"Hey, Barney!" He'd stop what he was doing and start slowly across the field toward the person doing the calling. Somehow he knew he was not the only one wanted; he'd stop and check out the whereabouts of his charges, and if they were not following he'd go back to them and in some manner let them know they were to follow. And they did.

His companionship was not limited to weanlings. Occasionally Woodhill would get in a lay-up off the track, and Barney would be its attendant until it settled down. He'd also help with fillies off the track, those that had been retired and were entering the broodmare ranks. I don't recall Woodhill ever having a filly with a let-down problem, which I'd see frequently everywhere else, and the only apparent difference was Barney.

And he was invaluable when trying to load balky horses. He'd go anywhere you led him—into any kind of van or trailer—and more often than not other horses would follow him. Anyone who ever had a skittish yearling to ship had to appreciate that.

But old Barney had not taken this last winter well. He had begun to look his age. He was moving slower and his old backbone was sagging. Now Whitey said he was not getting around well, and his eyesight was becoming suspect.

Whitey pulled a slip of paper out of his pocket and handed it to me. I read it:

Dr. Kendall,

Please put Barney to sleep. I think his time has come.

Estelle Wharton

"I hate this, Whitey," I said as I tucked the note into my pocket. "This is probably the sweetest horse that ever lived."

"I know, Doc. That's why Rufe ain't here. He's had that note the last two or three times you've been here and he keeps saying he forgot. Mrs. Wharton insisted today."

"What are you gonna do with him?"

"We'll bury him out back. A hole's already been dug."

"How are you gonna get him back there?"

"The wagon's hooked up to the trailer out back."

"Whitey, he weighs six hundred pounds. You'll never get him up on that thing."

"We're way ahead of you, Doc. Take a look."

I walked out the rear of the barn and there was the tractor and flatbed wagon. Leaning against the wagon were four or five long 2×12s, forming a ramp at about a thirty-degree angle from the ground.

"We'll walk him right up there. He'll go anywhere you lead him," explained Whitey.

"I guess there's nothing to do but get on with it, then," I said. "Go ahead and get him on the wagon. I'll get the stuff."

James, the kid who worked in Barn 3, put a shank on Barney and took him out of his stall as I went back to my car. On my list of favorite things, euthanizing anything comes just below having my teeth pulled with pliers.

I took the bottle of euthanasia solution from my trunk and got a needle and syringe. I drew enough for a 600-pound horse into the syringe and noticed there was only a small amount left in the vial, not enough for another horse, so I pulled it into the syringe, too. I looked at it and saw that it was about a 750- or 800-pound dose. With normal medications, I'm very careful to use the correctly calculated dosages, but somehow I didn't feel an overdose here was particularly danger-ous to the patient. Overkill was not a worry.

I went out behind the barn, and there were Barney and James up on the wagon. As I walked up the ramp, I noticed Whitey's eyes were a little moist. He saw me looking and turned away. He said, "I'll go get the tractor keys. You go ahead." And he walked into the barn.

"The keys is in the tractor," James whispered after Whitey left.

I patted Barney's old head a couple of times. "Old boy, I'm sorry, but I guess it's necessary." I was choking up a little, too.

The injection was quick. He went down almost before I could get the needle out of his vein. I waited a couple of minutes and checked his palpebral reflex. None. He was gone.

Whitey came back out. He spoke to James. "Pull his halter. Mrs. Wharton wants it." Then to me: "Rufe needs you over at the mare barn." He acted angry.

I drove over to Barn 2. Rufus didn't mention Barney or ask how things went. We very solemnly went through and checked several mares. It was April, the middle of the breeding season, and checking mares was what I did most. In addition, one mare in the barn had had her foal die after a dystocia and had developed a particularly nasty mastitis. She took quite a while this particular day, and all in all, we were probably at Barn 2 for forty or forty-five minutes. Rufus never once mentioned Barney.

After finishing everything, I was putting things back in my car and going over the follicles of a couple of the mares with Rufus. As we were talking, Whitey and James drove by on the tractor, heading to the rear of the farm. They should have dumped their load by now, I thought, instead of just heading back with it.

Rufus stopped talking and stared at the wagon with its unhappy cargo. I could see the tears forming.

"Doc, I never felt so bad about anything in my life," he said.

The wagon was about fifty feet past us, heading by on the main farm road. I started to agree with him, but before I could speak, Barney lifted his head.

This wasn't possible! I'd given him a 20 to 30 percent overdose of the most potent euthanasia solution available. I'd checked his palpebral reflex. He was dead!

"Stop!" I shouted, and ran toward the wagon as Whitey put on the brakes. Rufus was right behind me.

I hopped up next to Barney just as he rolled up on his belly. He looked over at me and gave a very drunken nicker.

"Rufe, he's alive!" I yelled.

For the first time since I'd been on the farm that day, Rufus smiled. "I'm no vet, Doc"—he beamed—"but I think you're right!"

The old pony was struggling to get to his feet now. Rufus told Whitey to pull the wagon over to the loading chute. Barney's halter was gone, so Rufus looped the shank he was holding around Barney's neck and guided him gently off the wagon. He staggered badly.

"Doc, I ain't gonna let you do this again," Rufus said. Whitey and James were smiling as broadly as he was.

If they had headed straight back with the wagon when I'd left Barn 3, Barney would have been in the hole and covered up by now. They explained that the tractor wouldn't start and they'd had to call Willie, the farm's mechanic, to get it going.

"Is Mrs. Wharton in the house?" I asked. They said yes, so I told them to put Barney back in his stall. I wasn't about to try again.

I drove on back to the house. A couple of extra cars were there, but company or not, I needed to speak with Mrs. Wharton.

She answered the door with very red eyes and handkerchief in hand. Behind her were her daughters, Cynthia and Claudia, both with tears streaming down their faces; theirs were the extra cars. Barney's demise had brought them together to share this most unhappy time.

"Is it over, Dr. Kendall?" Mrs. Wharton asked.

I told her what had happened. I don't recall ever having made three women so happy at one time, or even at three separate times.

That was a few years ago. Barney still doesn't get around too well. He still doesn't winter too well and spends a lot of time inside in cold weather. He still bumps into things sometimes, so he's in a small, treeless paddock with a quiet old ex-racehorse gelding as a buddy.

I asked some other veterinarians if they'd ever had a euthanasia failure. None had. I checked to make sure I hadn't accidentally used a bottle of solution that had expired, but it was still well within date. I called the drug company and asked if anyone else had reported a problem. No one had, but they suggested that perhaps the vial had become contaminated from a previous use, thereby reducing its effectiveness. I don't believe that was the case, but I can't say for sure. All I know is that Barney didn't stay dead that April day several years ago.

And no one has asked me to put him down again.

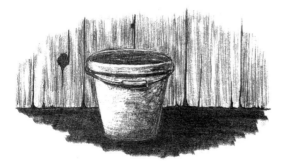

PSYCHOLOGY

I once did quite a lot of racetrack work, but I found I wasn't really suited to it. There are several reasons, among them: (1) lamenesses often remained a mystery to me no matter how diligently I searched for the causes; (2) I never understood why a horse had to be trained in the middle of the night (what was wrong with nine A.M.?); (3) I disliked trainers who had me worm five horses during the day and then would ship out overnight, payment having slipped their minds; (4) holding horses together for "one more race" was preferred to actually trying to heal or cure them; and (5) many trainers preferred to let the veterinary needle try to take the place of proper training and/or race selection. The racetrack was a frustrating place for me, but it was also a place to meet potential farm clients, and in that respect was very helpful.

A vet working the tracks does not wait to be called; he makes the rounds of the barns on the backstretch every morning and checks with his regular clients to see if anyone needs anything or has any problems. Most trainers begin their training days between five and six in the morning, so the vets usually show up by six-thirty. Personally, I think that's ridiculous, but Granddaddy sent 'em out early, and horse racing is a tradition-oriented business.

When I was working the tracks, I was young and eager. I usually showed up by six or before so I would be there in case some trainer needed a vet early, before his regular vet showed up.

I didn't really dislike track work, but as I said, it was frustrating. A couple of examples of item (5) above—one justified, one not— stand out.

≈

Marcus Jefferson is retired now, but when I was doing track work he trained a few horses that he also owned. The horses were cheap, and both they and Marcus had limited ability. Victories were few and far between. Mrs. Jefferson ran a small neighborhood diner, and the word was that her income was the only thing that kept the racing stable afloat.

Marcus never had a regular veterinarian. Whoever was around when he needed one was who he used, so I would always stop by his stable a couple of times each morning and usually two or three times a week he'd have some work for me. And he always paid—an excellent but far from universal trait among trainers.

I mentioned that Marcus had limited ability as a trainer. This was no secret. The word around the backstretch was that if Marcus had trained Man O'War, that great horse would never have won a race. That was probably a slight exaggeration.

After a few weeks around the track, I realized why Marcus's ability was so limited: He was lazy and he didn't know his horses. He frequently failed to exercise his animals properly, so they weren't fit for their races. Occasionally one of his horses would be claimed, and in every case the horse would run better for the new trainers than it had for Marcus. He bemoaned his bad luck that the horse would finally "develop" just as he lost it, but everyone knew it was simply a matter of more conscientious training.

In saying Marcus didn't know his horses, I don't mean he couldn't tell them apart. He knew that Falcon was the bay gelding, that Queenie the Rose was the chestnut mare with the white face, that Prissy Princess was the chestnut mare without the white face, etc. But he *didn't* know, for instance, that Falcon wanted to go longer than the six-furlong races Marcus continued to put him in. When Falcon was claimed, his new trainer began running him at a mile-and-a-sixteenth and a mile-and-an-eighth, and the old boy responded with two wins and two thirds in his first four starts.

And Marcus didn't know that Queenie the Rose was hurting. It turned out to be an osselet in her left fore ankle and I was the vet who found it, and if *I* found it, it had to be pretty apparent.

Eventually, Marcus realized that he was missing things and decided to do something about it. But what he chose to do did not involve more careful observation. He chose to cover his mistakes with drugs.

Some medications are permitted in racing, although which ones vary from state to state. Any legal drug administered must be reported by the vet to the state racing commission, a ruling designed to prevent the owner and/or trainer from overdosing a horse and, theoretically, assuring that the medication given is actually needed by the horse.

One morning as I passed through Marcus's area, he called me over. "Doctor," he said (he never called me or anyone "Doc"), "I got Prissy Princess in tomorrow night. I want you to come by in the morning and medicate her."

"Medicate her?" I questioned.

"Yeah. Bute, Lasix, some kinda steroid."

Bute is a pain-reliever permitted by many states. Lasix, a diuretic, is also allowed in many states; it is used in the cases of exercise-induced pulmonary hemorrhage—bleeding from the lungs—a fairly common problem in race horses. Steroids are pretty much not allowed, although some will not show in post-race tests.

"Golly, Marcus," I said, "why do you want bute and Lasix? She's not a bleeder, and she doesn't seem to be hurting. And you know I can't give her steroids."

"Dr. Ferguson and Dr. Walinski can. Why can't you?"

Remember, I was young. And naive. I knew certain drugs wouldn't test, but I never dreamed a licensed veterinarian would possibly ever even *consider* giving them to a horse entered in a race. I was shocked and didn't know what to say, so I went back to the other drugs he'd asked for.

"What about the bute? She's not sore, is she?"

"No, I don't think so," Marcus admitted. I'm sure that was true. He wouldn't really have known.

Wayne, the kid who helped him, was with us. "Wayne, is Princess sore?" I asked.

"Don't think so, Doc."

I turned back to Marcus. "Then why do you want to give her bute?"

"Well, Doctor, if she does have a problem we don't know about, bute'll help it."

I shook my head. "And the Lasix? She's not a bleeder, is she?"

"I don't think so."

"Wayne, have you ever seen any evidence of bleeding?"

"Never seen a drop," Wayne replied.

"Then why, Marcus?"

"Maybe she's bleedin' inside," Marcus reasoned.

"Marcus, I can't give bute and Lasix to your horse if there are no indications for them. There's no justification. I mean, she just doesn't need medicating, so it won't help. You don't take an aspirin if you don't have a headache."

He stared at me blankly. "Yeah, sure, Doctor. I understand. What about steroids?"

"I can't give her steroids. It's against the rules. You know that."

The next morning—the day he wanted the medications—Marcus didn't need me to do anything. The morning after that I looked in the paper to see how Prissy Princess had done the night before. Seventh in an eleven-horse field.

I went by Marcus's barn. He was on the track with a horse, so I spoke with Wayne.

"How's Princess?" I asked. "She ran up the track."

"She's okay, Doc. Just slow."

"Does Marcus understand that all those drugs wouldn't have done any good?"

"Don't think so. Yesterday morning he had Doc Ferguson look at her. He gave her five shots."

Bute and Lasix were two of them, I was certain. The other three? I don't know. One was certainly a steroid.

Marcus never asked me to work on any of his horses again.

Wallace Givens was a contemporary of Marcus. Wallace is now sending his charges to the Big Oval in the Sky, but back then he was a living trainer. He had been a jockey in his youth but outgrew it and turned to exercise riding. When age became a factor, he became a trainer. Wallace wasn't a bad trainer nor was he good, and the horses under his care were also neither good nor bad; he made ends meet but not by much.

Wallace hit a dry spell one year when I was doing his vet work. He had seven horses at the track, but one was confined to its stall with a foot fracture; the other six were sound and racing, but not too successfully. Over the three previous months the six had made a total of thirty-three starts, and only twice had any of them been on the board. None had won.

He tried everything. He tied tongues, he untied tongues. He put blinkers on, he took blinkers off. He put them on legal medications, he took them off legal medications. He shod them differently. He switched jockeys; he switched feeds; he switched bridles, bits, saddles. He had me do blood counts and he had me jug them. Nothing worked. They continued to run up the track.

One day he called me into his tackroom. I went in and he stuck his head back out the door, looked both ways, evidently saw no one, and closed the door. Then he locked it. There were a few small beads of perspiration on his forehead as he came over close to me.

"Doc," he whispered, "I gotta win a race. I'm gonna lose my horses if I don't."

I was at a loss as to what to say, so I didn't say anything.

Wallace went on. "You gotta help me, Doc."

"Wallace, I can't do anything. Maybe you should drop them down a notch."

"I can't do that. You gotta help me. Give 'em something."

"Give 'em what?"

"I dunno, Doc. *Something*." He looked around and lowered his voice even more. "Hop," he gulped.

"Hop!?" I said in a normal voice. Wallace winced visibly and held a finger to his lips. "Wallace, I can't hop your horses."

He pleaded on, but I stood firm, and he finally let me go.

He had a three-year-old filly in that afternoon, and she ran sixth, only beaten four lengths but sixth nonetheless. The next morning, as I entered his shedrow, he was morose.

"Doc, Mr. Morrison's takin' his horses," he told me. Morrison owned the filly that had run the day before and one other horse, a gelding that had also run sixth about a week earlier. "You gotta help me."

"Wallace, I can't do anything. Maybe they need a break. Maybe you should take 'em out of training for a while, turn 'em out."

He looked horrified. "I can't do that! I got bills! If they're turned out, I ain't gettin' paid!"

Two days later he approached me again. "Doc, I got Jivey in today. *Please* give him somethin'." It was a pathetic, lengthened "please," one that probably had four or five extra *e*'s in it.

Jivey was Jungle Jive, an older gelding that had had a little class in his youth but was now a mid-range claimer. The previous year he had won four or five races and brought home nearly $40,000, but this year he was oh for five and his best finish had been a distant fifth.

A brilliant idea struck me. I decided to show Wallace that "hop" wouldn't help his horses, that only proper training, conditioning, health, race selection, and genetic makeup would do any good.

"Okay, Wallace," I said in a whisper, "I'll help you." I looked around to make sure no one was near and then pulled him into a stall. Still whispering, I said, "I'll give Jivey something, but no one must know. Understand?"

He beamed. He almost chuckled. "Oh, thank you, Doc! Thank you! Nobody'll hear anything! Oh, thank you!" I was afraid he was going to kiss me.

I told him I'd be right back and went to my car. I drew two cc's of sterile normal saline into a syringe and held the clear liquid up to the light. "It needs some color," I said to myself, and then drew one-tenth cc of vitamin B_{12} into the syringe. B_{12} is red, and this less-than-a-drop made the mixture in the syringe a delicate, very pale pink. Neither the saline nor the B_{12} would have the slightest effect on the horse; in fact, the race wasn't until midafternoon and it was now about seven A.M., so the stuff wouldn't even be in the horse's system by race time.

I placed the syringe in my shirt pocket and went back to Wallace. "Let's go see Jivey," I whispered.

Junior, Wallace's assistant trainer/groom/hot walker/stall mucker/gofer, was with Jivey. "Send him somewhere," I whispered.

"Junior, go get us a bucket of hot water," Wallace ordered. Junior walked off.

We went in the stall. I pulled the syringe of pink liquid out of my pocket and showed it to Wallace. His eyes got big. "Wow!" he gasped.

"Check outside the stall," I directed. "Let me know when it's clear. I don't want anyone to see this."

Still wide-eyed, he gulped and nodded. He stuck his head out the stall door and looked both ways. "Not yet, Doc," he said in a whisper. A hot walker led a horse by. "Okay, now!" he said.

I injected the harmless fluid into Jivey's jugular vein. "There you go, Wallace. If this doesn't help, no drug will."

Wallace was sweating. He was shaking. "And it won't show, Doc?"

"Not a trace," I assured him.

I couldn't charge him for this. After all, I'd used less than a nickel's worth of "medication" that would have no effect on his horse anyhow. "Wallace," I lied, "I can't charge you for this. If anyone ever saw a ticket on this, all hell would break loose."

With somber seriousness, he replied, nodding, "I understand, Doc. But don't worry. I'll take care of you."

Jivey would lose again, I believed, and Wallace would see that "hop" didn't help and he'd go back to his training methods. Eventually his cold spell would end.

Jungle Jive was in a $10,000 claiming race that afternoon, down from $12,500 in his previous start. He was 15 to 1 in the morning line, but the bettors didn't think he looked even that good. He went off at 32 to 1, the second-longest price on the board.

And, unfortunately, he won. Easily. Six lengths.

Nothing showed in the post-race tests, of course. Nothing was *there* to show.

The next morning Wallace was walking on air. As I entered his shedrow, he called to me, "Doc, I got somethin' for you!" He handed me a $5 win ticket on Jivey. "I wish I'd a bet 50 for you," he said.

"Me, too," I agreed, and thanked him. Somehow this hadn't worked out exactly as planned.

A few days later he had Regal Mike, a three-year-old colt, in. This colt had been okay at two—a couple of wins—and had won his first time out at three, which, until Jivey, had been Wallace's last victory. Since then, Mike had managed only a third in his last six starts.

On the morning of the race, Wallace dragged me into his tack-room and asked for some more "hop." Well, why not? I thought. It doesn't hurt anything, it makes Wallace feel better, and maybe he'd see *now* that it doesn't help, so I gave the colt the two cc's of pink liquid in the same furtive manner I had used with Jivey.

Mike went off at 14 to 1 and lost by a nose in a photo finish. Again Wallace was ecstatic, and this time he had bet $10 across for me.

Enough, though. No more. He had to learn he was doing it on his own merits and that of his horses.

Two days later he ran Ladybelle, a five-year-old mare—as sound as a dollar but oh for her last eight. She had once run successfully for as much as $15,000 but was now down to $7,500.

Wallace asked again for his "hop." "I'm out of it," I told him. He looked as if I'd said his daughter had run off with a 300-pound Hell's Angel named Shark.

"Doc, you can't be! You can't be! What'll I do?" I thought he was going to cry.

I told him I was sorry. He mumbled something about scratching Ladybelle, but ended up running her. Thank heavens, she won. At 10 to 1. He didn't have any tickets for me the next day, though.

Wallace's luck had evidently turned around, but he kept asking for the "hop" and I kept telling him I couldn't get it and he kept on running without it. His horses began winning every fifth or sixth time out, and even Morrison brought his two back to him.

Every once in a while he'd ask me if I'd been able to get his "hop," and I finally told him it was no longer being manufactured, which was true because I had been the one "manufacturing" it.

"Too bad," he sighed.

Yes, it was too bad. I had enjoyed cashing those tickets.

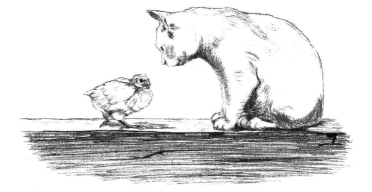

HOLLYWOOD

.

The racehorse industry attracts people with money. Because of this, those of us plain folks in the business probably have a little more contact with celebrities than most plain folks. Even so, up until I was into my thirties the only celebrity I'd ever known wasn't a celebrity yet when I knew her.

Her name was Sally Masterson, and you're right—you never heard of her. We were classmates in high school and we dated a while, but Sally was a very pretty girl with Hollywood aspirations, and that's where she headed soon after graduation.

And she made it, more or less. Not as Sally Masterson, though. She changed her name, appeared in a few movies and eventually became a TV actress. She was in a short-lived sitcom series several years back and frequently appeared as a "guest star" in other series and made-for-TV movies. I haven't seen her in anything for a number of years now, so I assume she has retired.

A lot of people have told me that women age faster than men, but that simply isn't true. Sally and I are living proof. When her series was on, her age was mentioned in an article in the newspaper. At that time I was forty-two. When we dated, Sally was one day older than me, so it seemed that she, too, should have been forty-two. Miraculously, though, the paper said she was thirty-six. Obviously, I was aging at a far faster rate. (More than a decade has passed since and I have not seen her age again. I have often wondered if she has ever reached forty.)

But as I said, that doesn't really count as knowing a celebrity. The first real contact I had with celebrities who were celebrities when I met them occurred when a client of mine with a very picturesque farm was approached by a movie company. They wanted to use his farm in the filming of a movie about a race horse.

And what a plot! A crippled foal is born and no one wants him. The decision is made to put him down, but the owner's daughter won't allow it. She takes the foal and raises him and trains him and he turns out to be a champion. Happens every day. But I figured if they had wanted my opinion of the plot they'd have asked for it and they hadn't, so I didn't say anything.

I didn't know all this was going on, though, until one summer morning when I showed up at the farm to remove sutures from a cut on a mare's shoulder that I had repaired nine days earlier.

When I drove up to the main barn, I saw about a dozen vehicles and various strange people milling around.

Carlos, one of the farm's employees, was waiting for me. He hopped in the car with me and said, "Doc, she is in the back barn. I go with you to hold her."

"What's going on here, Carlos? Who are all these people?"

"The movie people."

"What movie people?"

"Don't know."

When we reached the back barn, there was a message for me to stop by the office on my way out. Removal of the sutures took all of two minutes, and when I reached the office, Lester Rhodes was there.

"Hi, Lester. What's this movie stuff?"

"That's what I wanted to see you about. They need a vet."

"But what's happening? What's the movie?"

"Where have you been? It's been in the paper and on TV for days."

Maybe so, but I hadn't seen the paper, and TV newscasts are boring. He explained the whole situation to me. The title of the movie was *The Thoroughbred,* and his main barn and grounds were being used. His house, a Southern mansion type, was going to be used for exterior shots.

"They need a mare lying down to look as if she's foaling," he said. "They asked me if I knew how to make a mare lie down, and that's when I told them they need a vet."

"It sounds pretty hokey, Lester. Who's in this thing, anyhow?"

"I've never heard of most of the cast, but the guy playing the farm manager is Steven Richards and the farm owner is Marjorie Fallon."

He went on to say he had told them I could anesthetize a mare for the foaling scene.

"What mare?" I asked.

"Dolly."

Dolly was an old Quarter Horse mare who served no function, but Lester liked her, so she stayed. I laughed. "I look more like a Thoroughbred than Dolly does," I said.

"No one will be able to tell when she's lying down. Do you want to do it?"

I said sure, then I followed him over to meet the movie people.

Before we go any further, let me tell you about the two actors he'd mentioned. Steven Richards was great for the part of the horse farm manager, I thought. I had never seen him in any role other than that of a cowboy. He had guest-starred on every TV western ever made, and he'd had his own cowboy series several years back.

Ruggedly handsome and outdoorsy, he looked as if he had been born in the saddle.

And I'd always liked Marjorie Fallon. I remembered her in movies all the way back to my childhood. First she had been a kid sister, then the romantic lead in B movies, then a mature sophisticate, but she had always been pretty—blond, blue-eyed, slender. Now she was evidently going to be the mother of an almost-grown daughter. That probably put her near fifty, I figured.

When we reached the main barn, Lester introduced me to two people, a man and a woman, the names and titles of whom I didn't recall for two minutes. One was an assistant something and the other was his or her helper—in other words, an assistant assistant.

"Dr. Crandall . . ." the woman began.

"Kendall," I said.

"What?"

"Kendall. My name is Kendall."

"Kendall Crandall? That's an odd name. Okay, Kendall . . ."

I started to correct her, but she kept on.

"Now, Kendall, we need a horse to lie down. That's the way they give birth, right?"

Before I could agree or say anything, the guy started talking. "You see, Kenneth, the animal needs to be . . . Here, I'll show you." And he motioned for me to follow.

"Where's that big stall?" he hollered. I assumed he meant the foaling stall, and I'm sure it was right where he'd seen it last, but I let a young man with a three-foot-long ponytail show him.

"This is the door," he said, pointing to the door, "and we want the animal to lie down over there"—he pointed to the far right side of the stall—"with its rear toward this—the door." He showed me the door again.

"The 'animal' is a mare, and she's a *she*, not an *it*," I said.

"No problem," he said.

"Can you make the animal lie down like he described?" asked the woman.

I assured her that I could. "When do we do this?"

"We'll get all the farm scenes done early. Be here Friday at nine," she commanded.

"What if I have another appointment Friday at nine?" I didn't, but I might have. She looked at me as if I had burped, then looked at the guy.

"We're on a schedule, Kent," he said as if he were speaking to a slow six-year-old.

"Okay, Friday at nine. Before I go, how do I bill this?"

"Bill!?" he said, and looked at the woman.

"We plan to credit you as 'technical adviser,'" she said.

"How much will that get me at the grocery store?" I asked. "I'll need to be paid."

They looked at each other. "Present your bill Friday," he said.

Friday morning at eight-forty I pulled up to Lester's barn. I walked in and there were dozens—literally—of people there. I saw Carlos.

"Doc," he said, "this is stupid. None of them knows nothin', but I got Dolly here." He pointed to a stall, where the old mare was quietly chewing on some hay.

"Well, Carlos, it won't be long. They told me nine o'clock."

Then I saw the woman assistant-whatever.

"Hi," I said. "I'm here and ready."

"Who are you?" she asked.

"The vet. Kendall Crandall."

"Oh, yes. Dr. Connell. Sorry. We'll be a little while. Take a seat and we'll call you when we're ready."

Take a seat, she said. There were no seats. Then halfway down the barn aisle I saw an empty canvas chair next to another one in which a man was seated. I went down to it and asked the guy, "Can I sit here?"

"Help yourself," he said, and I sat down.

I looked at him more closely. It was Steven Richards.

"Who are you?" he asked.

"My name is Grant Crandall—I mean, Kendall—and I'm a vet here to make a mare lie down."

"Steve Richards," he said, offering his hand. " I hope you've got a lot of time."

"Why?"

"This is the most fouled-up outfit I've ever worked with in a life-time of working with fouled-up outfits. Everything is about a day behind and lagging and we haven't really even started yet."

"Shoot, I have an eleven o'clock appointment."

"Go ahead. They won't know you're gone, and they won't miss you. You'll be back in plenty of time if you don't return until tomorrow."

"Can I sit around and watch for a while? I've never seen a movie being made."

We talked for about half an hour, then someone called, "Steve! Where are you?"

"Down here," he called back.

"Who's this guy?" I asked, as a youngish, very slightly built man trotted down the aisle toward us.

"He's the guy with the crayon," he replied.

"What's he do with a crayon?"

"He colors in the bald spot on the back of my head." He turned his back to me. "See? The lights shine off it otherwise. We're shooting the scene where I tell the farm owner her best mare's just had a crippled foal."

"They haven't shot the scene where the mare foals yet. Shouldn't that come first?"

"It will in the movie."

The young man stood behind us, coloring on Steve's head with a brown marking pen. He looked at me. "Are you in this scene? I'll need to do you, too."

That hurt. Yeah, I knew my forehead was a little larger than it used to be, but I didn't know my scalp was showing through in the back, too.

"No," I said, "I'm a technical adviser."

Steve spoke. "There's the star." He pointed down the aisle. There was Marjorie Fallon and another woman. "I guess it's time."

"Can I watch?"

"Sure. C'mon. Just stay out of the way."

We both stood up at the same time. He was short! This was Steven Richards, tough-guy rugged cowboy hero! He was about five-eight! He'd been the same size as everyone else in the westerns I'd seen him in, and in his own series he had been bigger than everyone else! I didn't know what to say, so I just followed him.

And there was Marjorie Fallon. She was as blond and as beautiful as she had been in any movie. And she was tiny! Five-one would have been stretching it. Ninety-five pounds, soaking wet.

The other woman was actually a girl. She looked to be eighteen or nineteen. I don't remember her name—I'd never heard of her before—and she was playing the part of Marjorie's daughter. She was smaller yet. Where's Dorothy and Toto? I thought; I've found the Munchkins.

In looking back now, I can see Sally Masterson. When we dated, the other kids teased us. I was six-two by the time I was sixteen, and Sally was more than a foot shorter than me. I remember seeing her in films, and no one had been more than a few inches taller than her. It hadn't occurred to me before. I wondered if you had to be small to act, but then the scene began. It went something like this:

> (*Steve walks out of a stall, drying his hands on a towel. Marjorie and the daughter walk up.*)
>
> MARJORIE (*in a concerned tone*): We were out to dinner. We just got the message that Princess Athena foaled.
>
> STEVE (*dejectedly*): Yep. 'Bout an hour ago. Doc Walters just left. He says he's a cripple—epiphysitis. He'll never race.
>
> MARJORIE (*shocked*): My God! I won't raise a cripple!
>
> DAUGHTER (*pleadingly*): Oh, Mother, you can't put him down. Princess Athena has been so good to the farm over the years!
>
> MARJORIE (*heatedly*): We don't stay on top by raising cripples! Call the vet back! (*She turns and storms out.*)

Dr. Walters, the vet in the script, was evidently pretty sharp. It seems he diagnosed uncorrectable epiphysitis in a foal less than an hour old. Moreover, this was a condition I'd never seen in a newborn foal. In fact, until that point, I'd never even *heard* of it in a newborn foal! I was impressed.

I was enjoying this. While they repeated the scene, I went to the car and called my eleven o'clock appointment. It was routine stuff; they said I could come on Monday.

It was after ten-thirty. I found the woman assistant. "How long before we lay the mare down?" I asked.

"Please be patient, Dr. Cummings. It won't be long."

I went back and sat down. Steve came over and sat down, too.

"They've got something else on tap, but I'll tell them we need to do the foaling scene, if you like. Otherwise you'll be here all day and maybe it still won't be done," he said.

And he did. There was some confusion, and it took nearly an hour for them to prepare, but finally some guy yelled out, "Where's the animal?"

"I have her, señor," Carlos called.

"Oh, hell. Where'd we get the wetback?" a man standing near me said.

"He's a naturalized citizen, jerk," I said.

"Who the hell are you?" he demanded.

"I'm here to make the mare lie down, if it's any of your business," I told him.

He turned his back on me and walked away.

"Who's that?" I asked Steve.

"The director," he answered.

"He's a jerk," I said.

"Grade A," he agreed.

I had already gotten the drugs I needed to anesthetize Dolly, and I was ready. To no one in particular, I said, "You'll only have about half an hour after she goes down before she'll start to wake up. Don't dawdle."

From the stall she'd been in, Carlos led Dolly down the aisle toward the foaling stall. Just before entering the stall, she stopped and urinated. She'd evidently been holding it all morning; it was magnificent! It looked like gallons as it splashed all over the clean blacktop of the barn aisle and splattered on the shoes and pantlegs of those standing near.

"Oh, shit!" wailed the director.

"No, that's urine," I corrected.

Carlos led her into the stall as the woman assistant ordered someone to clean up the urine. But Dolly wasn't finished. Just inside the stall, she defecated. This, too, had apparently been held for some time. It was a pile of which to be proud!

"Oh, shit!" howled the director again.

"That's right," I said.

No one seemed to know what to do about this. After a minute, Carlos handed me Dolly's lead shank and said, "I be right back," and proceeded to remove the pile of manure. No one thanked him.

Dolly's anesthesia went smoothly. Carlos held her where I told him to, and I injected the drugs. Within thirty seconds she was lying there, zonked.

"Okay," I said, "you can shoot your scene."

Steve came in the stall rather tentatively, I thought. "Is she good and out?" he asked.

"Oh, yes, she's as under as she can get."

He walked in carefully, keeping a safe distance from the old mare and eyeing her suspiciously. He was afraid of her! The cowboy was afraid of horses!

I didn't want to embarrass him, so I sat on Dolly's hip and patted her on the rear. She didn't budge. Steve came over near her.

"All right, you two get outta there!" someone barked, obviously meaning Carlos and me. We left the stall. Steve knelt near Dolly's rear.

I don't think anyone said, "Lights! Camera! Action!" but someone did say something, and the filming began. Steve was kneeling there behind Dolly, and a little old guy in coveralls walked into the stall. I had noticed him before standing around doing nothing. From the look in his eyes, I thought he might be drunk. Now, though the look in his eyes was the same, he had a stethoscope around his neck, a little black bag in his hand and a hand towel hanging from a rear pocket. By golly, I thought, this must be Dr. Walters!

The scene proceeded along these lines:

ACTOR PORTRAYING DR. WALTERS *(as he enters stall)*: Well,
    Johnny, it looks like you've done a good job.
STEVE *(looking up and smiling)*: Not my first one, Doc.
DOC *(bending over where Steve is kneeling)*: Let's check this little
    fellow out. *(He puts the stethoscope in his ears and listens to an
    imaginary foal. Then, in a very serious tone)* I don't like the
    looks of this, Johnny. This colt has epiphysitis!
STEVE *(alarmed)*: Oh, no! Don't tell me that! This is Princess
    Athena! The farm's counting on this colt!
DOC *(standing up)*: I'm sorry. He's a cripple. He'll never race! *(He
    takes the towel from his pocket and wipes his hands.)*

They did the scene two more times, but I don't know why. It
looked and sounded the same to me each time.

By the end of the third take or whatever it's called, Dolly's anesthesia was wearing off. Although she still didn't move, she snorted a
little. Steve jumped and Dr. Walters flew out of the stall.

In redoing the scene three times, I began to see where I had mis-
understood the method of diagnosing epiphysitis in a newborn. Being
a condition of the legs, I had always thought that I had to look at the
legs, see the foal get up and move around, possibly even touch the
affected area, maybe take X rays. All Dr. Walters had to do was listen
to its heart and lungs while it was lying down and not moving. I was
impressed. He was *good!*

There was also his declaration that the colt would never race.
Wow. I usually had to wait months, at least, to determine that.

One thing I didn't understand, though. He hadn't touched anything except his stethoscope. Why, then, had he dried his hands? Did
he have a wet stethoscope? This question remained unanswered.

Dolly was waking up. She had rolled up on her chest and was
looking around groggily.

"Okay," said a woman I hadn't seen before, "get her out of here."

"We can't yet," I told her. "It'll still be a few minutes before she
can stand and several more before she'll be ready to walk."

"We need her out of there!"

"I'm sorry. It'll probably be another six or seven minutes."

"They won't move the animal!" she yelled to the woman assistant-whatsis. She came over.

"Dr. Connors, we're through with her. You'll have to remove her now." She was serious.

The discussion continued, and as it did, Dolly got up. Carlos hooked the shank to her, but she wasn't quite ready to walk. Lady assistant pointed out that she was now up. I agreed with her. She insisted, for a minute or two, that we get her out of there. By this time Dolly had come together, and Carlos walked her very slowly out of the stall, out of the barn and on toward the back of the farm. The two women gave each other looks confirming that they had won; the horse had been moved at their insistence.

While I had lady assistant's attention, I asked how I should bill this. She again told me that I would be credited as "technical adviser," and I again told her that I needed money. She said to turn my bill in to her, which I did immediately.

She looked at it. "Who's Grant Kendall?" she asked.

"Me," I said.

"Then why did you say your name was Keating!" It wasn't a question, so I didn't answer.

As I began to leave, I saw Steve sitting back in his chair. I went over to him.

"Steve, I'm leaving now. I enjoyed meeting you."

"Hey, you know what?" he said. "I was amazed at how you handled yourself around that horse. They scare me to death."

"Then why do you play cowboys?" I asked.

"I look like one. And the pay's good."

We shook hands. As I turned to go, I saw Marjorie Fallon down the aisle talking to Dr. Walters. "Introduce me to her?" I asked Steve.

"Sure. Hey, Marjorie! Come over here! I want you to meet a guy!"

She turned from Dr. Walters and came over, smiling broadly.

"Marjorie, this is Grant Crandall. He's a horse doctor."

I started to tell them it was Kendall but thought better of it. Marjorie offered her hand. "Dr. Crandall? I'm very happy to meet you, and I must admit to a great deal of respect. Horses scare me to death." She was well into her forties, but beautiful. And tiny! Fine bones, small delicate features. I had rarely seen a woman as pretty in person. Even though she had a few years on me, I wondered what her marital status was, but then I remembered mine. Just as well. I left then.

The filming evidently moved right along, because in less than a month the whole crew was gone, not only from the farm but from the state as well. I kept expecting a check, but it never came. The movie was released several months later. I went to see it, not for its artistic value but to see the credits. I thought maybe I'd be listed as "technical adviser" after all, in lieu of being paid.

I wasn't.

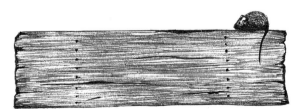

Part Three

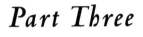

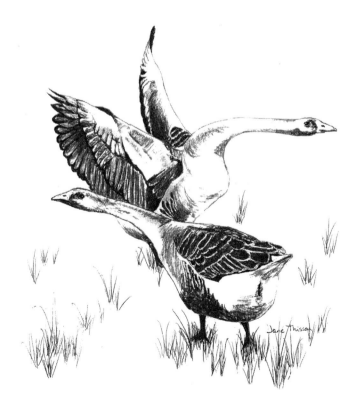

GUS

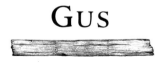

One morning I went to the pond with a little corn to feed the ducks. Scrooge was gone by this time, and little Daisy—all her children, grandchildren, etc., were much bigger than she was—was getting slower and never left the barn anymore except to meet me about twenty feet in front of the building when she heard me coming.

This particular morning was unusually foggy for central Kentucky. It wasn't a world-class fog—I've been in fogs in San Francisco and London where you couldn't see out of your car window—but it was dense enough to cause the local residents to talk about it all day and was probably good enough to cause a few minor fender-benders before it lifted.

The ducks knew I was coming, even if they couldn't see me very well. It was that time of morning, and besides, I called them: "Ducksducksducks! Ducksducksducks!"

I was spreading the corn out amidst a chorus of quacks and peeps, depending on the age, when I saw in the mist what appeared to be two very *large* ducks. They were about fifteen feet away, and I could just make out their silhouettes.

"Who are you guys?" I asked, stepping a little closer, and tossed some corn in their direction.

They walked away as I approached—not fast, but fast enough to maintain their distance from me. Obviously they were strangers. The resident ducks *never* retreated—they liked their corn too much.

"Okay, guys," I said. "I'll see you later when the fog's gone." And I turned to go back to the barn.

"Honk!" someone said.

"You're geese!" I exclaimed. "Well, welcome! You can stay as long as you like."

"Honk!" they repeated.

I finished feeding the horses—or at least I think I fed the horses; it was difficult to account for everyone in the fog—and went back to the house.

"Guess what," I said to no one in particular, "we have a couple of Canadian geese out there on a layover."

The kids wanted to go see them right away, but my wife said, "Isn't this an odd time for Canadian geese to be migrating?" It was July.

That hadn't occurred to me. Of course, Canadian geese wouldn't be going north *or* south in July.

"Gee, that's right," I admitted, "I couldn't really see them too well—I just assumed they were Canadian geese."

I had nothing scheduled that morning, so about an hour later, after the fog had lifted a little, we all went out to see what we had. There were two very large, very white domestic geese in the center of the pond.

"They sure aren't Canadian," I said.

"Where did they come from?" my son asked.

"I guess they walked over here from a neighbor's pond," I said. "Does Mr. Clark have geese down there with his chickens?"

"I don't think so," answered my wife. "I don't think he has anything on his pond."

"How about the Averys behind us? They have a big pond."

I didn't know the Averys except to say hello to him if I saw him somewhere. I didn't even know what his wife looked like, but my wife had been invited over there once or twice.

"I have no idea, but I'll call and ask," she offered.

And she did. No, the Averys had a few ducks but had never had any geese at all.

She called Mr. Clark. Another no. We called around the area, asking neighbors. No one was missing any geese; indeed, no one even owned any geese.

Well, we assumed, they flew in. I had a real hard time with that, though; these birds were huge, and I didn't think they'd be very good flyers. (I think I was right; I have never seen them fly in the many years they've been here.)

Their origin was a mystery that has never been solved, but they were here to stay. Neither was particularly afraid of people, so they must have been around humans at some point. They kept a slight distance for a few weeks, then started coming up with the ducks whenever the corn bearer appeared.

We called them Gladys and Gloria. Gladys was the larger and more outgoing of the two, frequently walking from the house to the barn with me, honking all the way. Gloria, on the other hand, rarely left the pond and was not very vocal.

Gladys loved the baby ducks. There would be two or three hatchings a year (we give *lots* of baby ducks away) and Gladys would accompany the mother duck and her ducklings until the babies got pretty big. She would even sit with them on the nest sometimes. The mother ducks seemed to understand that she was helping.

When the babies went to the pond, Gladys would swim in the rear of the group, making sure all the babies stayed together.

Gloria, however, seemed to have no opinion one way or the other concerning the ducks or ducklings. She minded her own business and expected them to mind theirs. She and Gladys were nearly inseparable at the times when Gladys was not working as a nanny.

These were good geese, loud but kind. I remember being chased by a pair of geese my uncle had when I was three or four years old. One of them caught me and bit my heel, and it hurt! Uncle Frank told me that was the nature of the birds.

But Gladys and Gloria weren't like that. I was a little apprehensive at first about the kids being around them, but neither one ever did more than hiss occasionally.

They had been here three or four years when one winter morning I went to the pond and found Gloria lying limp in the water. She was dead.

I took her out of the pond and couldn't find a mark on her, so I put her in a plastic bag and took her to the university animal pathology laboratory, where they could do a postmortem examination on her. It may just have been old age, but it could have been some disease brought in by wild ducks, and I didn't want all our birds getting sick and dying.

It wasn't either, however. She had cancer, a tumor on her right ovary. They said they'd never seen one in a goose before, but I suspected their exposure to dead geese ranked down there with their exposure to dead rhinos, so I don't really know how rare Gloria's tumor was. It was interesting, though.

Over the next few weeks, Gladys spent less and less time at the pond and more and more time at the back door, waiting for someone to come out. I realized that, like Daisy years earlier, she was lonesome for her own kind, but a goose sitting on your doorstep is not something you want. I think if Gloria's passing had come in the summer when baby ducks were hatching, Gladys wouldn't have taken it so hard, but it didn't and she did.

And a full-grown goose on your doorstep is not a good thing. Because she spent so much time there, she would eliminate there. Geese make *huge* piles and it was necessary to clean up after her twice a day. My wife was threatening to look into the making of pâté de fois gras if something wasn't done.

Well, once again a client came forth to help.

Fred Ballunger owns a small farm about five miles from us and has a pond full of ducks. Most of his ducks are descendants of Daisy and Scrooge, but he also has some he purchased to introduce some fresh genes.

Fred's pond is about twice as big as ours and far prettier. Ours is out in a field; Fred's is in his yard, which looks like a park—everything is trimmed and manicured right down to the water's edge. I mow my grass once every couple of weeks unless I can get out of it. Fred mows his at least twice a week unless he thinks it should be done more often.

One afternoon a few months after Gloria died, I was at Fred's place checking a foal born that morning. As we were finishing—everything was fine; he was a big, healthy, ornery colt—a goose walked into the barn.

"Where did that come from?" I asked.

"Some folks down the road had him as a pet but he got too big, so they brought him here and asked if I wanted him," Fred explained. "The only problem is, he won't go near the ducks. If they're on the pond, he leaves. I think he's lonely for another goose."

I told him of Gladys's loneliness and our problem at the back door.

"Well, he's yours if you want him," he said.

I went home and got the trusty plastic pet carrier and headed back to Fred's to claim the goose, which I had already named Gus. In my mind, I was picturing a relationship somewhat like that of Daisy and Scrooge, culminating in a lot of baby geese. What fun that would be!

This tale, however, does not have a happily-ever-after ending for Gus and Gladys. In fact, Gladys plays little part in it from here on out.

Gus was easy to catch. He was still in the barn when I got back to Fred's farm, and Fred just walked up to him and picked him up.

He did voice a little displeasure when we put him in the carrier, though. It wasn't tall enough for a goose of his stature, but he scrunched down and we closed him in.

I took him home and toted the carrier down to the pond, where Gladys was swimming—one of the few days she wasn't hanging around the back door. She came out of the water when she saw me, probably expecting some corn.

I set the carrier down and said, "Look what I've brought you, Gladys." I opened the carrier's door and Gus stuck his head out and looked around.

After maybe two minutes—it seemed like an hour—he finally crept out and walked around. Then he headed over toward Gladys. Ah, love, I thought.

He stretched out his wings—they must have been four feet from tip to tip—and honked two or three times. Some goosey small talk, I imagined.

Then he put his head down, beak straight forward, and ran at poor innocent Gladys, who hadn't made a sound. He bit her twice very quickly, and she headed to the water. Gladys was larger than Gus, but aggression often makes up for size.

Next he proceeded to chase any ducks that were nearby. These were all Pekin/Mallard crosses, remember. Mallards, of course, fly very well, but I don't think Pekins fly—Scrooge never did, anyhow—and these hybrids all flew very poorly, if at all.

The poor ducks didn't know what to think. Our dogs had never bothered them and Cat, the mighty huntress, had seemed to know she should leave them alone, even in her kitten-producing days.

There was considerable flapping and quacking as they all headed for the pond. Pretty soon Gus was the only bird left on the bank. I think Fred's interpretation was wrong; it was *not* that Gus wouldn't go near the ducks; instead he chased them away from him.

Well, I thought, maybe it's just a period of adjustment. I myself was always kind of shy and aloof when I was with a group of strangers, and since I was aware that that kept me a stranger perhaps longer than I should be, I could relate. However, I didn't walk up to the strangers and punch them all in their noses, which was, in essence, what Gus was doing.

But eventually I would get acquainted with the strangers and even occasionally make a friend or two. So would Gus, I was sure.

And that's right. I was sure. I was sure *wrong*. In time Gladys and the ducks learned to go where Gus wasn't. I had to spread the corn far and wide at feeding time because Gus would forgo eating to chase and bite the assembled ducks if I fed them in a small area, as I had done before. Poor Gladys left the back door out of self-preservation; the only place she was safe was in the pond.

Eventually everything settled down. Gladys had her ducklings in the summers and the ducks had each other. And Gus had himself by his own choice.

In Gus's third summer of residence with us, he made his most serious error.

He bit *me!*

It was a hot afternoon, and I had put on shorts after I finished my vet work for the day. Laurie had gotten married and quit, and the horse population on the farm was down, so I had begun doing all the work myself, with the aid of a little forced child labor. It was feeding time, so I walked up toward the barn. About halfway there, Gus came to meet me.

"Hi, Gussie," I said, and walked on by him.

"Honk!" he said, and spread his wings a little.

Then he bit me in the back of my poor bare right leg. Doggone, it hurt!

I turned and kicked at him, missing by two feet and succeeding only in kicking off the canvas loafer I was wearing. It went about twelve or fifteen feet down the gravel drive and I lost my balance. In catching myself, I put my right foot down hard on the gravel, jabbing several sharp little rocks into my bare sole.

Hobbling after my thrown shoe, I snarled at Gus, "Do that once more and you're outta here!"

"Honk!" he reiterated, and headed for the pond.

I was pretty careful around Gus for the next few weeks, and I warned the rest of the family to be on their toes, but there were no incidents. Every once in a while, Gus would extend his wings slightly, but that's as far as it went. I attributed his attack to the fact that maybe he had had a bad day; I think we're all guilty of that now and then, although most of us don't physically attack anyone. After a couple of months it was all but forgotten.

Then one morning I was in the feed room gathering the grain for the horses. I had two buckets and opened the feed room door to take them out to the two yearlings that were in stalls.

And there was Gus! He was in the center of the barn aisle—and his wings were spread wide, his head was down, his beak was straight forward, and he was heading for me!

I jumped back in the feed room and slammed the door. After a minute I opened it a crack and peeked out. He was still there! I grabbed a handful of corn and tossed it as far down the aisle as I could while still maintaining the door as closed as I could.

Gus went after the corn. I waited a second and then opened the door to go out again. I was no more than three feet into the aisle when he saw me. He stopped eating and came at me again.

I got back in the feed room just in time—I heard his beak hit the door. I was trapped. It was late August and school had just started, so the kids were gone. My wife had gone off somewhere early to do something, so I couldn't even call for help.

Gus stayed there by the door for nearly half an hour. Every time I peeked out, he'd spread his wings, hiss and lower his head. I guess he got bored with it, though, because I finally saw him, through the feed room window, strutting off toward the pond. When I was sure he was far away, I ventured forth and fed the horses, who were not thrilled with the lateness of their meal.

To this point, I was the only one to have seen Gus's aggressiveness toward people—or person, I should say. Neither my wife nor the kids had been attacked, so when I told them of my harrowing experience and narrow escape, they weren't totally believing. In fact, I think I detected strong disbelief.

I was extremely wary for the next several days, but nothing untoward occurred. And for many days Gus didn't even come to the barn.

On one of these days when he wasn't around—or so I thought— I came out of the barn with two buckets of grain for the horses in the field. As I got ten or twelve feet from the barn into the wide open spaces, where there was no protection, he came at me from around the corner of the building, wings out, head down, beak out, hissing!

I jumped aside, and he missed me on the first stab, but then he came right back at me. I swung a feed-filled bucket at him and connected on the side of his head, knocking him for a loop.

This made him mad, and he got up and came at me again. I kicked him in the side just as he bit my bare leg. The kick knocked him back and away from me, but he had my skin firmly in his beak and he tore it open.

I guess the kick hurt him because he just sat there—or maybe he'd fulfilled his goal of drawing blood. Whatever, he got up after a few seconds and headed on back to the pond.

When I got back to the house, I challenged my wife. "There!" I cried. "Now do you believe he bites?!"

My wife glanced casually at my mutilated leg. "It just looks like a scratch," she stated calmly. "Believe who bites?"

"Gus!" I shouted. "That miserable, rotten man-eater out there!"

I still didn't think she believed me. "If he's so mean, why doesn't he bother anyone else?" she asked.

That was a good question, but not one I spent much time on. I was too busy trying to figure out why I had married for love. If I wasn't going to be believed and sympathized with, I might as well have married for money.

Gus seemed to be a more reasonable bird after our latest altercation. I was very careful whenever he was near, but he acted like his old self. It was not until many weeks later, close to Halloween, that he attacked again.

I was coming out of the barn, and he came at me. I used a bucket again, but he just came back for more. I kicked him and then ran for the house. He chased me for about thirty yards before he quit and ambled over to the pond as if nothing had happened.

I knew that trying for my family's sympathy and understanding was a lost cause, so I didn't even mention this attack. And as before, Gus settled down for a few more weeks.

The next assault occurred just before Christmas. He got me from behind, in the fleshy part of my thigh—and even though I had on long pants, that one really hurt! It happened like before: He came at me from around the corner just as I was leaving the barn. I would have wrung his neck if I had caught him; he must have realized that because he ran to the pond as fast as his little legs would carry him.

I suggested to my wife that we have roast goose for Christmas dinner. She thought I was joking.

The periodic attacks continued for the rest of winter, through spring and into the next summer, and I was still the only one he chose to pick on. I was possibly a better person for it—my awareness of my surroundings and reaction time both improved drastically.

If someone was keeping score, I was probably leading by a two-to-one ratio, if we based the score on the number of times he actually got me.

Finally, he made a serious error: He let someone see an attack.

While I was at the barn, a very important long-distance call came for me. My wife said I'd call right back and she came to the barn to get me. She was about fifty feet from the barn when I came out and Gus zoomed out from around the corner in attack mode.

"Look out!" she yelled.

But I was ready. I was *always* ready these last few months!

I swung a bucket and he ducked. I missed, but so did he. I ran and he came after me. As I ran past my wife he was gaining on me, but when he saw her he stopped. He just plain stopped! Just like a kid acting up in school when the teacher suddenly appears. Then he strolled off nonchalantly to the pond.

"Now do you believe me?" I gasped, trying to catch my breath.

"If that's what's been going on, why don't you get rid of him?" she asked.

"I offered him for Christmas dinner," I reminded her.

"I don't mean 'get rid of' as in 'kill,' I mean 'get rid of' as in 'give away.'"

"Whom do we dislike enough to wish him on? Other than your brother?"

She didn't deny this last part. "He doesn't have a pond. Put an ad in the paper."

In the relatively rural Kentucky county in which we live, our local newspaper is a weekly freebie that consists of news about rezoning hearings (which are invariably denied, successfully keeping us in the nineteenth century), announcements of engagements, pictures of local residents with the large or odd-shaped pumpkins or cucumbers they've grown, and ads. Lots of ads. "Will watch children in home." "Free kittens." "For sale: brass bed and pair of women's shoes, size 8D, never worn." "Free kittens." "For sale: 1957 Rambler. Make offer." "Free kittens."

I personally never thought anybody ever answered these, but my wife assured me that they did. "There wouldn't be so many in it each week if they didn't get results," she reasoned.

So I called the paper. It came out on Mondays, and this was Thursday.

"I'd like to place an ad," I said to the voice on the other end of the line.

"What you want it to say?" asked the voice.

"Goose. Free. Come get him." And I gave our phone number.

"Okay. Be in Monday. Bye."

On Friday afternoon the phone rang.

"You the one with the goose?" a female voice asked.

"Yes, ma'am," I replied.

"We'd like him but we can't get him 'til my husband gets off work. It'll be around eight before we can get there."

"He'll be here." I gave directions to our place. Then I said, "The paper won't be out 'til Monday. How do you know about him?"

"I work at the paper. We've wanted a goose for the kids for a long time."

"This goose is mean," I warned. "He bites."

"Oh, that's all right. We still want him."

Okay, she'd been warned. He was theirs.

A little before eight that evening, a pickup truck containing a young couple and two small children drove in. They had a large cage in the bed of the truck.

They introduced themselves—Joe and Sally Stallings—and asked where the goose was. We went to the barn and he was there waiting. I told Joe he'd have to catch him and explained why I wouldn't get within ten feet of him by choice.

He walked toward Gus. "Be careful," I warned.

Gus stood there and let Joe pick him up. He allowed himself to be carried to the cage in the bed of the truck. Their kids came around to pet him.

I told them again, "Be careful," as Gus rubbed his head against Sally's hand. They gave me a distrusting look.

"Does he have a name?" Sally asked.

"Gus," I said.

"Oh, great!" squealed their little girl. She was probably seven. "That's what we wanted to name him!"

"They had decided on Gus on the way over here," Joe said.

"What are you gonna do with him? Is he just to be a pet?" I was visualizing the headline in the newspaper, right next to the picture of the fourteen-pound tomato: "Goose Eats Local Family."

"We're gonna put him in the fair," said Sally. "They have a Dressed Poultry contest and the kids are gonna make an outfit for him. He'll be so cute!"

I couldn't picture Gus being "cute," nor could I picture Gus allowing himself to be dressed up. I could, however, picture still another headline, right next to the announcement of Earline Earlywine's engagement to Bobby Don Fryman: "Goose Runs Amok at Fair."

Gus *won* the Dressed Poultry contest. The headline, next to the picture of the old fellow with his potato that looked like Mickey Mouse, read, "Goose Best Dressed," and there was a picture of Gus in a coat and hat along with Joe, Sally and their two very happy children.

A few weeks later Joe called me. When I heard his name, my heart sank. I figured he was going to tell me Gus had bitten off someone's finger or eaten a neighborhood child, but neither was the case.

"This is greatest pet we've ever had!" he exulted. "Do you know where we can get another one just like him?"

And I had thought the problem was with Gus. I guess it was me all along.

THE FOUNDLING

It was Christmas day, but that never mattered to horses. I think it may be their way of getting even for a perceived slight about two thousand years ago. In all the manger scenes I've ever seen, there are cows, sheep, camels, donkeys, even a dog, but *no horses*. I think that the choice of December 25 for many horses to get sick or hurt is not coincidental.

You can buy them calendars and circle the day in red and tell them *not* to do anything to call attention to themselves on that day, but it just doesn't do any good. If they acknowledge the calendar at all, they do so by eating it.

Ben Wickersham was the resident vet on one of the country's largest Thoroughbred breeding farms, and each year he would try to take the last two weeks of December off to head down to Alabama with his family. That's where both he and his wife were from.

But in his absence, the horses on Sawbuck Farm still needed veterinary care and this is where I came in. The workload of an equine veterinarian is usually pretty slow at the end of the year, so I covered for him in his absence. It gave me something to do and it allowed him to get away, so it worked out well for both of us.

I wasn't wild about the Christmas Day stuff, however, and it always happened. At least one horse somewhere would need my attention, but usually it was two or three, and they were always at various extremes of my practice area.

This particular Christmas morning I had received only one call. A mare at Sawbuck had aborted overnight. Moreover, she had been sutured and had torn badly.

Before going any further, however, let me say that at the time of this story Sawbuck Farm had been around for nearly forty years and had grown to some 5,000 acres divided into three separate tracts. One tract was a training center, one was for weanlings and yearlings and the third—the main farm—was for stallions and mares.

The stallion population varied from year to year, but usually there were about twenty. Stud fees ranged from $500 up to $100,000 or more.

The farm owned more than three hundred mares, but the quality was not as wide as that of the stallions; nearly all of the mares were very high-class runners and/or producers.

On the main farm were Stallion Barns A and B and Broodmare Barns 3 through 22. I assume that Stallion Barns A and B were once called Barns 1 and 2 because there were no Barns 1 and 2 on the place. They were numbered logically; Barn A was the first one you encountered on entering the farm and Barn B was right behind it. By following the farm road, you came to Barn 3 about a quarter mile away, and as you drove deeper into the farm you would come upon Barns 4, 5, 6 and so on. By the time you got back to the upper teen-numbered barns, you were way into the 3,500-plus acres that made up the main farm.

This particular Christmas morning, Chris Woodside, the assistant farm manager of Sawbuck, called around six-thirty.

"Doc," he began, "I'm real sorry to call you on Christmas, but a mare slipped this morning. She needs attention, but I think she can wait a little while if you want to open your presents first."

I thanked him for his consideration and told him I'd be there in about an hour and a half. Then we let the kids wreak havoc unwrapping their gifts. Around seven-forty I left my wife to assemble toys and insert batteries and headed off to Sawbuck.

Chris had said Barn 21. The higher the number of the barn, the less that went on there. Most of the barns had from sixteen to twenty-four stalls, and with three hundred mares there were very few horses beyond Barns 15 or 16. I had never been as far back as 21 before, and when I got there I found it to be an old twelve-stall barn that housed four late-foaling imported mares. They would be moved farther forward as their pregnancies progressed.

The mare that had aborted was named Esmeralda, and she was from Chile. She had been one of the last mares bred the previous breeding season, her final cover coming on the third of July (the final day the breeding sheds were open was the fourth).

Most mares, even sutured mares, aborting before six months would not tear much, if at all, but Esmeralda, evidently realizing that I needed something with which to occupy my day, did a bang-up job of splitting open. She tore in a V, sideways through the suture line and up around both sides of her rectum. Repair was no big deal but it would be a little time-consuming.

As I replaced her divots with the aid of the skeleton holiday farm work crew (Chris was holding her tail, and normally the assistant farm manager would *not* be a tail holder), the kid who had driven the muck wagon out to be dumped came into the barn.

"Mr. Woodside," he said to Chris, "there's a horse out there."

Chris looked at him. "Billy, this *is* a horse farm, you know."

"Yessir," he replied, "but I don't think this one belongs."

"Is it loose?"

"Nossir, it's in a paddock."

Chris told him he'd check it out as soon as we finished with Esmeralda. That took another ten minutes, and then Chris and I chatted a little as I cleaned my instruments. Billy stood by, fidgeting nervously.

Finally, he said, "Mr. Woodside . . ."

"Oh, okay, Billy. Sorry. Show me this horse that doesn't belong."

"It's out back here," he pointed, and led the way. I went along.

About forty feet behind Barn 21 was a large, long hedge, broken by a gap about ten feet wide through which an old, unused path ran. This is apparently where Billy had taken the muck wagon to dump it; there were fairly fresh tractor marks in the grass.

Billy led us through the gap, and behind the hedge we found a small paddock, smaller than two acres.

"Look there," said Billy, pointing to a horse in the paddock.

"Horse" is what it was, but barely. Standing in the middle of the paddock was a veritable scarecrow of a horse—a tall bay with prominent hip bones and all ribs and backbone showing beneath a weather-beaten hide, and a long, matted mane. It didn't have a halter.

"Holy cow!" exclaimed Chris. I agreed.

"Billy," Chris continued, "run to the barn and get a halter and shank."

Billy trotted off, and Chris and I entered the paddock. The top hinge on the gate came loose from the rotted wood and the gate fell over rather than swinging open. The horse raised its head and looked at us, then drooped its head again. We walked toward it, and it just stood there. Chris bent down and looked under the animal's belly. "Doc, this is a stallion!" he announced.

I had been looking around the paddock. It was winter so there would be no real grass, of course, but even considering that, this place was terribly overgrazed. There was an old metal water tank—empty. The bottom was rusted out. "Chris," I said, "there's no water in here."

He looked around, too. "There's no water and there's nothing to eat. He must drink from there." He pointed to a small ditch running through the far (low) end of the paddock. He was probably right; water would run through there when it rained or after a thaw.

"And look at those feet, Doc." All four hooves were horrible—in some places there were two-inch-long pieces of hoof sticking out, and in others the hoof was broken off to nothing.

Billy returned with the halter and shank. The horse didn't move as Chris slipped the halter over his nose and buckled it by his left ear. He hooked the shank to it and began to lead him toward the gate.

The horse followed along slowly—very slowly—but he did follow. It took about five minutes to get the fifty or sixty yards to the barn. Chris placed him in a stall and told Billy to toss him a flake of hay. The horse dived into it.

Jerry, the young man working in the barn, gaped at the sight. "Gee whiz, Mr. Woodside, where did that come from?"

"I have no idea, Jerry, but I'm sure gonna try to find out."

Chris had been employed by Sawbuck for about two and a half years. He had been hired when old Mr. Henderson had retired. Mr. H, as everyone always called him, had been the manager for years, and on his retirement Roger Mitchell, who had been Mr. H's assistant for about three years, had been moved up to manager. As so often happens, Mr. H passed away within a few months of his retirement. Chris said this was the first year since he'd been employed there that they'd had horses as far back as Barn 21.

"Doc," Chris said, "he needs something. Go ahead and do what you want. I'm going to call Roger and see what he knows about this." He went to his truck to call the farm manager from his mobile phone.

I had Billy hold the horse and I drew a couple of blood samples. The hay intake had stirred a little gut activity, and he passed a few small, hard, dry fecal balls. I picked up a couple in a plastic sleeve so I could examine them for parasite ova. Being certain he was full of them, I decided to worm him with a mild paste wormer. He was a tall horse, over sixteen hands, and should have weighed 1,200 pounds but I estimated his weight to be closer to half that. He was so thin and emaciated that the outlines of the bones in his legs and skull were evident. In order not to cause an intestinal blockage by dead parasites, I only gave him a 400-pound dose of wormer. He could have more later.

Jerry brought a bucket of water.

"Pour out about three-quarters of that, Jerry," I directed. "We don't want him to have too much too soon."

The horse inhaled it and went back to his hay.

Chris came back. "Roger doesn't know anything about this guy. He said he'll be right over." Roger lived on the farm, so it wouldn't take him more than ten minutes to get there.

I told Jerry to give the horse another quarter bucket of water. He inhaled that, too. He was inhaling his third quarter bucket when Roger drove up. Billy tossed him another flake of hay.

"Merry Christmas, everybody," Roger said. "What do we have?"

Chris told him all we knew. Roger looked at the horse.

"That is one sorry-lookin' critter," he said. "I think the last time we used this barn was the year before Mr. H retired. I guess that's three or four years ago. I don't know why a stallion would be back here."

"Is he a teaser, you think?" asked Billy.

"Yeah, probably," Roger answered, although I thought he was awfully large for a teaser.

Horses that race have the inside of their upper lips tattooed for identification purposes. Chris checked this guy's lip. "No tattoo," he said.

When the farm office opened the next day, Roger and Chris checked the records of the teasers. Sawbuck kept records on everything. The farm had five teasers at that time because of the large number of mares they had, and the records on these five were there, as well as the records of over a dozen other teasers the farm had used previously.

If the teaser was no longer in use, the record was noted with the final disposition of the horse: "Died" and the date, or "Sold" and the date, or "Donated" and the date.

On the records of two there were no exact final dispositions. On one it said "Retired" and was dated fourteen years before, but it didn't say what was done with him on his retirement. He was a bay Thoroughbred cross named Armor, and he would have been over thirty at this point.

On the other, the record said nothing. He was a bay Thoroughbred named Sorby, and he would be twenty now. The last recorded entry on his record was when he had been wormed five years before. Our horse must be Sorby.

Evidently when Barn 21 had last been used, the horse had been put back there to tease the mares. And when the mares moved out, he was just forgotten. For five years he was on his own in an overgrazed, underwatered paddock hidden behind a large hedge behind an unused barn.

One possible explanation for the forgetting of Sorby: Except in management positions, horse farms have a large and sometimes quick turnover of employees. The person in charge of Sorby may have quit or been fired on the day Barn 21 had been taken out of use five years before.

Just in case Armor was still around somewhere, Roger assigned a complete search of the back half of the farm. No other lost horses were found.

Old Sorby, if that is indeed who he was, responded well to a little TLC and groceries. Ben Wickersham took over his veterinary care a week later, of course, but he kept me posted on his progress. By spring he looked like a horse again. He was past his days as a teaser, but Roger and Chris figured the farm owed him something. He was moved up front to Stallion Barn B and given his own paddock. They treated him just as they did the valuable breeding stallions until he passed away quietly three years later.

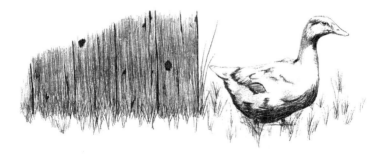

FANG

A great many things in life depend on perspective. There's the famous half glass of water, for instance: To a pessimist it's half empty; to an optimist it's half full.

Further, to Danny DeVito a six-foot-tall person is big; to Wilt Chamberlain he's not.

And so it is with old sayings and adages. Someone sees something and remarks on it, someone else hears and repeats it. Eventually, for want of proof to the contrary or simply because we *want* to believe, these things work their way into our everyday usage.

For instance, someone probably saw a cat climbing and performing various feats so well that he was moved to say, "As graceful as a cat."

And it caught on.

Suppose that same person saw a cat fall (or maybe he dropped it) and noticed that the cat landed on its feet. "Interesting," the guy thought as he picked the cat up and dropped it again.

The cat's opinion of these proceedings has not been recorded, but the person observed that ol' Tabby once again hit feet first. Thus, "A cat always lands on its feet" began its way into our consciousness and everyday language, and eventually, when someone had a setback but came out in good shape in the end, he "landed on his feet."

But it's all perspective, and the perspective here lies with the cat that was observed. With another cat, these faithful old sayings could have come out very differently. If our observer was observing a very large, very hungry cat, for instance, the old saying today may well have been "A cat always eats people who observe it"—that is, if the observer shouted it out to someone else just before the final swallow was made. It's not an adage likely to have great popularity or use in everyday living.

And, if the cat that was studied so carefully happened to have been Fang, the sayings would be more along these lines:

"As clumsy as a cat" and "A cat *never* lands on its feet" (or "A cat lands anywhere *except* on its feet").

Fang is a small orange cat, neither particularly handsome nor homely. Just an everyday-Joe sort of cat.

Some time ago my friend and client, Fred Ballinger, he of the ducks and parklike pond, called.

"Doc, you want a kitten?" he asked.

Fred had asked this question once before. A friend of his had one left from a litter and it needed a home. I told him we'd take it if no other home could be found. Obviously, on hearing this no further search was performed, so in a few days we had a half-grown, fully wild little female cat.

And she remained that way. Wild, that is. She grew. I think she's a very attractive cat, but I can't really tell. She's always leaving a room as I (or anyone) enter it. We named her Gary after one of my son's favorite baseball players, and she always avoided human or other animal contact. She gets along with our other two cats, Annie and Cat, simply because she never gets within hissing distance of either one.

"We really don't need another cat," I told him. "What's the story?"

"He's a stray in the neighborhood where one of the guys who works for me lives, and he's bothering the guy's wife," he explained.

I didn't understand so I said, "I don't understand."

"This kitten hangs around their door all the time and grabs at the woman. She's afraid it will hurt her. Unless he can find a home for it, he's gonna take it to the pound."

"What about you?"

"I've already got Corky and Nemo and the two barn cats. I just don't need another one."

That was true. Corky and Nemo were two very fat, very lazy house cats, and the two barn cats were equally fat and would probably have been equally lazy given the opportunity. Fred feeds well.

Knowing fully well what I was saying, I said, "If he doesn't find another home for it, I guess we'll take it."

And surprise! He called back two days later and said another home couldn't be found.

"Okay, Fred," I said. "How do I get this critter?"

"I'll have him here this afternoon. I'll have him in the house, but I won't be home. You know where the key is, so just come in and get him when you get the time."

This worried me a little. This kitten was terrorizing a woman and now Fred wasn't even going to be around when I came to get it.

Armed with the trusty pet carrier, I went over to Fred's that afternoon. I retrieved the key from its hiding place, pulled open the screen door and inserted the key into the lock.

And then I heard it! A bloodcurdling series of yowls, snarls, hisses and growls was coming from inside the house! Poor old Nemo and Corky, I thought—being devoured alive by this beast. I wished I had brought gloves. I knew this creature would shred my hands.

The thought occurred to me to leave and come back that evening when Fred would be home—I could tell him I hadn't had the time earlier—then he could catch and cage the monster. But too late! A girl who worked for him drove down the driveway and waved to me. He would know I'd been there.

Steeling myself, I unlocked and opened the door just a crack to peek in. Just inside, I saw Corky and Nemo. Their tails were erect, their ears were back and their hair was standing straight up, making them both appear twice their normal sizes.

And they were the ones doing the spitting and hissing and growling!

I opened the door farther and stepped in. There, on the couch, was a small orange kitten just sitting there. No hisses. No spits. No yowls. No growls. Just sitting there.

He was the size of a young kitten, maybe eight weeks old, but he had the facial maturity of one considerably older.

And he just sat there.

Have you ever seen strange cats when they meet? In a previous episode I described the interaction of Cat and Annie when they first met, a relationship that still continues after several years. Now docile, old, fat, lazy Nemo and Corky were acting like fierce jungle beasts—typical of a meeting of strange cats. I sometimes wonder why the species is not extinct.

And the newcomer not only also throws a fit, it usually hides as well. But not only was this little orange kitten *not* throwing a fit, it was sitting there in the open as if it belonged there and nothing was wrong.

Still wary, for I didn't know what had gone on before I arrived (maybe Nemo and Corky had had their rear ends kicked), I gingerly approached the kitten. He watched me advance cautiously toward him.

"Nice kitty kitty," I cooed, and slowly reached out with my right hand.

He eyed the hand and then sat up on his haunches, reaching out for me with his two front paws.

I pulled back. This terrorizer of women and animals was not going to get his claws in me!

He put his front feet back down on the couch and stared at me. Corky and Nemo were still throwing fits.

"Nice kitty," I murmured, and slowly placed the carrier on the couch and opened its door. "Nice, nice kitty." I reached ever so slowly toward him.

Up on his haunches he went, paws out. Back came my hand.

I was at a loss as to what to do. "A towel!" I said aloud. "I'll get a towel!" With a towel I could wrap him up and protect myself from his claws. I walked down the hallway toward Fred's bathroom.

There was no towel there. Fred keeps his home as neat as he keeps his grounds, and I doubt if a used towel was allowed to hang around very long.

I went back to the hallway and opened the first door I came to, looking for the linen closet. No, this was a coat closet.

Farther down the hall was another door. I tried it. No, wrong again. Books. Lots of books. I had never thought of Fred as a reader, but then, he probably never thought of me as being afraid of a kitten. One can never tell.

There were no more closets in the hallway and I didn't want to invade the bedrooms, so I ended my search for a towel and returned to the living room, where Nemo and Corky were still voicing their fear and disapproval of the interloper.

One was black and the other was gray and white, but even though I had known both for years, I never knew which was Nemo and which was Corky. It was sort of like bacon and eggs or Lum and Abner; they were always said together. "Corky and Nemo" or "Nemo and Corky." I had never had a reason to differentiate. (I *can* tell bacon from eggs.)

Anyhow, when I got back to the living room, the gray and white member of the firm had climbed the curtains adorning the front window, evidently in an effort to distance himself even more from the orange hellion that had been thrust into his environment.

I looked at the couch. The orange kitten was gone! That's why poor Corky or Nemo had taken to the heights, no doubt. Now I had to find where the beast was lurking.

(Later I realized that the reactions of these two intrepid felines might not have been a true barometer of the actual threat being made. In the normal run of things, the most fearsome object either Corky or Nemo ever had to face was the occasional catnip mouse.)

I got down on my hands and knees and looked under the furniture. "Here, kitty kitty. Nice kitty." He wasn't there.

I looked in the kitchen and dining room and back hall. I looked under things and on top of things and behind things. He wasn't anywhere. I had been down the hallway to the bedrooms and bathroom and he hadn't gone that way, I was pretty sure.

I searched again. I couldn't find him. The fact that he must have still been there somewhere was evidenced by the reactions still emanating from Corky and Nemo, but he was nowhere I looked.

The search went on for ten minutes or more, and finally I decided to give up and go. I would come back that evening and tell Fred the truth: I couldn't find the kitten. And that *was* the truth, if I omitted the first few minutes after my arrival, which I intended to do.

I closed the door on the pet carrier and picked it up off the couch. Something was wrong; it seemed to be too heavy on one end and it didn't hang correctly.

I looked inside through the bars on the door.

There he was—a little orange ball curled up asleep at the far end of the pet carrier. Asleep, he didn't appear to be too dangerous.

Well, I had captured the beast after all! Now to get him home in safety (mine) and hope he wouldn't be too hard on old Annie and the dogs.

He slept all the way home and was still asleep when I carried him into the house. Gary had been asleep on the footstool in the family room when I entered but immediately awoke and fled. Annie entered from another room and came over to where I had placed the carrier on the coffee table. She took one sniff, let out a low growl, put her ears back and began swishing her tail. I picked her up and put her outside.

When I opened the door, the dogs came in. They bounded over to the carrier, sniffed once or twice and began barking at it. They wouldn't hurt a cat—they had been raised with them—but they would bark at one. Of course, they'd also bark at lint or feather dusters or a rock they hadn't noticed before—they were nondiscriminatory in their noise-making.

I ran them back outside. I was going to let this little monster out and I didn't want to have to tend to scratched dog noses.

Okay, all the other critters were gone. My wife was out and the kids were at school. It was me against the orange bomb. One on one, the way nature intended.

I was afraid the combination of Annie and the dogs had gotten the kitten worked up, so before I opened the carrier door I peeked inside. He was still sound asleep! He hadn't moved. Lord, I thought, nerves of steel!

I opened the carrier door and stood back. I waited a moment but nothing happened. He didn't come out. I looked in. Still asleep.

I gently shook the carrier. No response. I looked in again. I was afraid he might have died or something. But I could see him breathing, so he was alive. I started to reach in and shake him, but thought better of it and got a yardstick to use instead. I could always get another yardstick, I reasoned, but hands were harder to come by.

I reached in with it and softly prodded him. He opened his eyes and shook his head. Then he reached out and laid a paw on the stick. I slowly pulled it back out of the carrier, and he followed its departure with his eyes.

I stepped back. The kitten stood up, stretched, yawned, then came toward the open door. He stuck his head out and looked around. Apparently seeing nothing to attack, he sat down. So did I, on the floor a few feet from the end of the coffee table.

I guess he caught sight of me at this point. He opened his mouth and said, "Anc!" A very harsh, metallic "Anc," at that. Then, still watching me, he stood up, stepped through the carrier door and began walking slowly toward me in what seemed to be a very purposeful manner. Stalking.

After a few steps he reached the end of the coffee table, but he kept on walking—right off the edge. He landed on his head. "Anc!" he repeated.

This move had not been a particularly graceful one, but I chalked it up to new environment, unfamiliar territory, stress, the car ride (although he'd been asleep and therefore unaware of the whole thing), etc. The fact that he landed on his head I attributed to all of the above plus the fact that the coffee table was very low and he didn't have time to get his feet under him before he reached the floor.

He got up, evidently none the worse from the fall, and continued toward me. I was beginning to feel that possibly this kitten was not the danger I had initially thought, but nonetheless I held out the yardstick.

He stopped and looked at it. He picked up a paw and slapped at it. Then he sat up on his haunches and batted it with both paws. He kept his claws in, I noticed.

I put the yardstick down. He watched it for a second, determined that it was apparently no longer going to play with him and then refocused his attention on me.

I was sitting cross-legged on the floor, and he walked over to me. "Anc?" he asked, then stepped up on my left knee, attempted to balance and fell off onto his side. A cat, when it feels itself slipping and/or falling, will dig in with its claws and try to hold on. This did not occur with this kitten.

Not totally sure I was out of danger but feeling fairly safe, I reached for him, carefully. He reached up and batted my hand, but did it gently and without extended claws.

I picked him up and carried him to the couch, where we sat for a few minutes. He was content to lie in my lap. Gary stuck her head in the room, saw that other living creatures were present and took off for unpopulated parts of the house. The kitten didn't seem to notice.

(I have often wondered what Gary does on those occasions when we have guests. Normally, we have four people in nine rooms, so she can pretty well avoid contact. Sometimes, though—usually holidays—we'll have guests, often as many as six or seven additional people. We don't even catch a glimpse of her at these times.)

I decided to call the kitten Fang. Any cat that can scare a grown woman and cause a vet to be uneasy deserved a fierce name.

I figured he might be hungry, so I took him to the cat food. It sits on a small table in the room I use as my office; if it were on the floor, the dogs would eat it. I placed him on the table and aimed him at the food bowl. He ate some but not much, but then, he wasn't very big.

I left him there on the table, which was maybe thirty inches high, and went about doing other things. After a few minutes I heard the metallic "Anc!" very loud and clear. I went to see what he was up to.

He was still there on the table, but not wanting to be. He was looking over the edge, apparently trying to summon the courage to jump.

He saw me come in. "Anc!" he pleaded.

("Anc," I am sure, is Fang talk for "meow." No one in the household has ever heard him say "meow.")

I tried to coax him down, but he wouldn't jump. This was going to be a problem; if the cat food was any lower, the dogs—big dogs—could get to it, but if one of the animals it was intended for couldn't reach it, that, too, would not be satisfactory.

We have a scratching post for the cats that is actually the trunk of a small tree. It's about eight inches in diameter and roughly twenty inches tall. I put it in front of the table on which Fang was stranded and gently pushed him off onto it. He sat there for a while, eyeing the still-distant but now closer floor, and finally decided to risk it. Gingerly, he slid off the post and onto the floor.

Eventually he learned to get to the food that way. He would carefully climb the post and then make the short hop to the table top.

Later that first day the family came home, and with them came the reentry into the house of Annie and the dogs. Annie hissed and snarled and growled and fluffed for two days. The dogs barked for two days. And for two days, while all this was going on, no one saw Gary.

But Fang seemed totally unaware. He'd watch them but go on about his business. If he found one of the dogs asleep, he'd bat her tail, but otherwise he seemed to pay no attention at all to any of the other animals.

He liked people. He would sit either next to or on someone whenever he could.

When he was on the couch, which was often, he'd frequently fall off and/or misjudge the floor. His head was his favorite landing site, but he'd also land on his tail or back or sides as well. I rarely saw him land on his feet.

At night he chose to sleep with my wife and me, but it was really with me. Or, more to the point, *on* me. If I was on my back, he'd be on my chest. If I was on my stomach, he'd sleep between my shoulder blades. If, however, I slept on a side, it was a much greater challenge to him. He'd try to sleep on my upper arm and shoulder.

This did not give him a broad base on which to relax, and I could feel the tension in his little body as he tried to balance.

I'm a light and restless sleeper, and I frequently shift positions many times during the course of a night's sleep. As I mentioned earlier, when a cat feels what it's resting on move, it will dig in with its claws in order to hold on or it will jump for safety. Fang never did either; he just fell off. If my shift propelled him toward the edge of the bed, he'd fall off the bed. We could always tell how he landed: A "clunk" meant headfirst, a "thump" was somewhere else. Rarely was there ever a "pat," indicating a feet-first landing. I worried about this for a while, but within seconds he was back on the bed and on me, so I stopped letting it bother me. He never seemed to suffer from the experiences, even though the most frequent sound was "clunk."

At my wife's urging, I took him to my small-animal friend to see why Fang was such a klutz. He didn't know, but he suggested that perhaps he had had an ear infection when he was younger and his inner ear was messed up as a result. Sounded good to me.

After Fang had been with us for a few weeks, he showed interest in going outside, so we let him out. Annie and the dogs had gotten used to him, so there was no danger. After an hour, however, my son called to me, "Dad, Fang's stuck in a tree!"

"That's okay," I answered. "Cats are always getting stuck in trees, but they usually get down just fine."

"No, come see—he's really stuck."

And he was. Somehow he had gotten his left hind leg wedged in a forked branch and he was hanging upside-down, frantically trying to grab the branch with his front paws. "Anc! Anc! Anc!" he screamed. I climbed up, unwedged him and carried him down.

It was a week before he asked to go outside again, and within a short time I heard my son yell, "Dad! Fang fell out of a tree!"

I ran to see. Fang was sitting there on the ground beneath a silver maple, shaking his head. "What happened?" I asked.

"I saw him sitting there on that branch"—my son pointed to a large limb about ten feet up—"and all of a sudden he started trying to grab hold with all four feet and then he fell. He landed kerplop on his back. Is he okay?"

I checked him over and he seemed to be fine.

Fang has grown to adulthood now. He never got very big; he may weigh six pounds, and an average adult tomcat probably weighs twelve. At one time or another he's fallen off everything he's been able to get on—tables, chairs, couches, beds, trees, fences, the scratching post. You name it, and if he got on it he fell off. Not every time, mind you, but often enough.

And usually he lands on his head. At least when we see him he does. When we're not with him, he may fall twenty times a day and land on his feet every time, but I doubt it. He says "Anc!" a lot.

It's probably good Fang wasn't around hundreds or thousands of years ago, back in the days of Old-Saying Creation. We might very well have a whole different outlook on life today.

And then there are the other old sayings, "As clumsy as an ox" and "Like a bull in a china shop." (I would love to have been there for that one.) After knowing Fang, I imagine somewhere there's an ox that can tap dance and a bull that drinks from a demitasse.

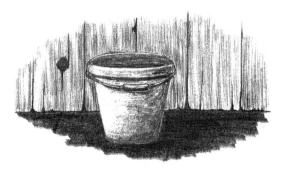

Señora

"Dr. Kendall, this is Sharon at Clear Valley. Mr. Anderson asked me to tell you that Señora's in season."

Rats.

Evan Anderson evidently didn't know how to use a telephone. During working hours, he always had his secretary, currently Sharon, call. As the farm secretary that was probably her job, but in the evenings and on weekends, if there was a need for a veterinarian, his wife or daughter would always make the call. In the middle of the night, if a foaling mare needed help, Robbie, the night watchman, would call. In eight years of working with Evan, the Clear Valley farm manager, he had *never* called me.

I understand Clear Valley's new manager, whatever his name is, is just the opposite; he maintains constant personal contact with his new vet.

That's one of the hazards of the job of equine veterinarian. A new farm manager—in an attempt to discredit everything his predecessor, no matter how successful, ever did—switches to his own choice of vet as soon as he takes over.

Evan and I, working together, had been very successful with Clear Valley's broodmares. In eight years we had averaged a live-foal crop of a little more than 90 percent from the farm's band of about thirty mares. In fact, the last breeding season that Evan was there, twenty-six of the twenty-seven mares conceived; it looked as if we'd maintain the 90 percent–plus average. But neither of us was there to see them foal.

I heard later from a young man who worked there that they only had twenty-one foals that next year, and in the yearling sales the following year, the Clear Valley consignment consisted of only eighteen head. Historically, the farm's entire crop had been offered for sale. It would be a lie to say that there was not a certain amount of satisfaction gained from seeing that everything had not gone well for them after my dismissal.

Clear Valley was a good account. An excellent account. The owner lived somewhere in Europe and only came to the farm about once a year. Absentee owners are the best kind.

One day, shortly after my final breeding season there had been completed, I went to the farm to remove sutures from a foal that had somehow cut its neck right above the shoulder. When I got there, the barn foreman said, "Doc, Mrs. Anderson wants you to stop by the house when you're done."

That wasn't a particularly uncommon message, although it was usually "Sharon wants you to stop by the office when you're done." It meant one of two things: Either my check from the previous month was ready or Evan wanted to see me about something. This time I had already been paid, so I thought Evan had something to discuss.

Removing the sutures was a quick process, once we got the foal down out of the rafters. He was one of those little guys that was evidently fine with one person, but associated more than one with unpleasant experiences. All of us—the foal, the barn foreman, the groom and I—lived through the suture removal, but it was nip and tuck for a while. Then I drove to the house.

"Hi, Rachel," I greeted Evan's wife. "Evan wanna see me?"

"I doubt it," replied Rachel, matter-of-factly. "He ran off with Sharon yesterday."

I thought she was kidding. I even laughed. But then I saw she was serious. They had gone the day before after work; he left a note, which she showed me, that said they were going to Florida, where he would train horses.

Evan was a good farm manager, but as a trainer he was sorely lacking. With him as trainer, Secretariat could not have won as a maiden claimer at a state fair. But obviously, that was neither here nor there.

I told Rachel I was sorry. I didn't know what else to say. I'd seen other people run off with someone, but I could always tell something was going on. With Evan and Sharon, though, it was a total surprise.

Evan was nice looking, I guess—I've never been a good judge of men's looks—and about my age—that is to say, not a kid anymore—and Sharon was very plain, although built like the proverbial brick chicken house (that's not a sexist remark, it's a statement of fact) and probably twenty-three years old, plus or minus. Rachel, on the other hand, was a very attractive woman who, if I hadn't been happily married, would have appealed to me far more than Sharon ever could. But I guess none of that added up to an unusual combination.

Rachel said she had called Mr. Moroni, the owner, in Italy or France or wherever, and told him of the turn of events. He had instructed her to ask me to continue doing the veterinary work as I saw fit. He also asked her to contact his local attorney and have him find a new farm manager.

The attorney was very efficient. He found someone within two weeks, and within three weeks Clear Valley was no longer one of my clients.

(Moroni gave Rachel thirty days to move, three months' salary [Evan's] and moving expenses.)

So much for the tale of woe. Let's get back to Señora being in season. This call came about two years before the change in management and in Sharon's first year with the farm.

Señora was Señora Sensi, a four-year-old mare that had won two or three stakes and more than $200,000 at two and three. A bone chip in a knee had caused her retirement in the fall of her three-year-old campaign, and she had been offered for sale privately by her owner. Evan had asked me to go to Ocala, Florida, to check her out, and at the last minute he'd decided to go with me.

As luck would have it, Señora was in season when we got to Ocala. It was early in November, and the farm manager said that was her first time to cycle since she'd come off the track eight weeks before.

I was able to do a full reproductive exam, including a culture, and everything was normal. The knee was X-rayed and the chip would never be a problem for a broodmare, so Evan bought her for Clear Valley. She shipped to Kentucky a week later and was put under lights right away.

Mid-February came and Señora had not come back in season, but that certainly wasn't uncommon. We waited.

By mid-March she still hadn't done anything. Evan was a little concerned, but he knew broodmares, so it was still no big deal. When she still hadn't shown anything by April first (we'd been specking her every other day for two weeks), we figured she needed a little help, so I gave her a hormone injection.

Ten days later, still nothing. Another injection. Still nothing. We began daily injections.

We were into May now, and by mid-May Evan was actively worried. "Grant, I spent a quarter million dollars of the farm's money and she won't even come in heat."

I shared his concern. After all, I had been the one who passed on her reproductive soundness.

Mr. Moroni, who rarely telephoned, was calling once a week to ask about her.

We went through ten days of progesterone followed by another injection of the hormone. Nothing happened. It was now early June.

Evan decided to just forget her now and we'd try her again the following year.

Then, on June 18, Sharon called. "Dr. Kendall, Mr. Anderson asks if you can come right away to check Señora Sensi."

I got there within the hour. It seems they had taken Peter, the teaser—if a person could get a dollar for every teaser named Peter or Dickie, he could retire in luxury—out to his paddock, and Señora, from fifty yards away, had come running to the fence, spraddle-legged.

They teased her and she was red hot.

I checked her and she was, indeed, red hot. She needed to be bred as soon as possible.

Evan asked my opinion. Would I breed a maiden mare so late in the season? I told him she had a good chance at a May foal if she conceived and there were a lot worse things than May foals.

He had gotten rid of the stallion season he had intended to use on her. He'd used it on a very old mare a few days before; he had intended to pass her because of her age, but because she had foaled so easily and had such a nice foal, *and* because he now had an extra season, he went on and bred her.

We went to the office, and Evan told Sharon to call around and see what was available and open right now. On her second call, she found an excellent young stallion that had been stopping his mares extremely well.

Evan got on the phone and spoke to the stud manager. He explained the situation and the quality of the mare and was told to bring her there immediately.

The next day I checked Señora again. She had ovulated. Everything looked pretty good.

But nineteen days later, the call that I began this episode with came. I got there and Señora was falling-down in love again. I specked her and her cervix was wide open.

"At least she's cycling," a disappointed Evan said. "We'll get her early next year." It was July 7, way too late to breed a maiden, even if the breeding shed had still been open.

I said, "We may as well culture her, just in case."

"Go ahead," he said.

The culture was negative, and Señora was put out with the only other mare on the farm that had no foal, another maiden but one that had been bred in early March and was in foal. Eventually Señora was put with the barren mares, an old mare that had torn badly and a middle-aged mare that had carried her foal two weeks over a year, not foaling until June. Technically, neither was barren because neither had been bred.

Summer and fall passed, and in late November Señora and her two companions were put under lights, along with a new maiden the farm purchased at the November sale.

The new mare was bred in February, on the opening day of the breeding season. The mare with the long gestation was bred a few days later and the torn mare in early March. Señora had not yet cycled.

"Nothing we did accomplished anything last year," I reminded Evan in late March. "I guess we just need to wait her out."

He agreed, muttering something about her ancestry and the price of Alpo going up.

In early May she was still anestrous. While I was checking a few mares, a new girl at the farm, Missy, said, "Doc Kendall, that mare there's in foal." She pointed to a paddock.

I looked where she pointed. "That's Señora, isn't it? No, Missy, she's empty. We cultured her last summer."

"I seen a lot of mares the last few years, Doc. She's in foal."

Evan walked up. "She telling you Señora's in foal?" He smiled.

I smiled back. "Yeah."

"Missy, look at her!" Evan commanded. "She doesn't have a belly or a bag or anything."

"I can tell by how she acts and moves. She's in foal!" She was adamant.

"I'll tell you what, Missy," I said. "Next time I'm here, I'll check her if it'll make you feel better." I smiled at Evan and he winked back. "Have her in the barn."

Nothing was going on at Clear Valley the next day, so it was two days before I returned. We had a ton of things to do—a couple of mares to suture, vaccinations and wormings for a few of the early foals, several pregnancy checks and palpations on mares either bred or to be bred, a culture on a mare that was back in season for the third time.

I arrived nearly an hour late, but I had called to warn them. My morning had started out with a colic, which had put everything behind. (In September and October, when equine vets are practically unemployed, I would welcome colics, but they always seem to occur when there's not enough time. That probably is a subparagraph under Murphy's Law.)

I got out of the car and asked, "Where shall we begin?"

Before Otto, the barn foreman, could reply, Missy said, "I got Señora up. Check her first." She pronounced it Sin-aura.

"There's too much to do and Doc's already behind," Otto told her.

"He said he'd check her!" Missy insisted.

I smiled at Otto. "Another few seconds won't matter now, and besides, she's right. I did say I'd check her."

Missy twitched Señora and stuck her rear out the stall door. Otto grabbed the tail and I stuck a lubed, sleeved arm in her rectum. I could only get in about eight inches.

"Holy cow!" I said. "Not only is she in foal, the thing's sitting right here!" I indicated a spot on the mare's side with my free hand.

"Well, damn," said Otto. "I better call Mr. Anderson." He went to the phone.

Missy beamed. "I told you she was in foal!"

Evan came right to the barn. He calculated her foaling date at around May 26 or 28, and it was already May 6.

"God, Grant!" he howled. "We've been feeding a jillion-dollar pregnant mare like she was barren! Moroni will have a fit!"

But Moroni didn't have a fit. He understood. Señora went on and made a normal bag and had a normal foaling on May 18, eleven months exactly from her breeding date. The foal was a normal, albeit small, colt, but he grew, and by the time he was ready to sell, his size was fine—smallish, but not little. He brought what they had paid for the mare, $250,000, and he went on to win a couple of stakes at two before he chipped a knee as his dam had done.

Señora was bred back on her foal heat and was as regular as clockwork until I was dismissed by the new farm manager. I assume she still is.

Evan was a flop as a trainer in Florida. Sharon eventually took off with someone else and he came back to Kentucky. He tried to go back to Rachel, but she told him to suck eggs. The last I heard, he had gone to California to train horses. Rachel got an uncontested divorce and married a banker. I hope she's living happily ever after.

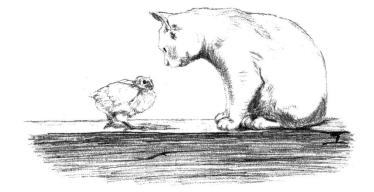

ANGIE

I don't like euthanasia, although sometimes it's the kindest thing to do. When I was asked to put Barney down, I felt it was necessary, even though it didn't take and everything turned out okay in the end.

I have lost clients over euthanasia. Once a client wanted me to destroy five (!) mares because he had had a little luck and was upgrading the quality of his stock. He didn't feel he could sell these five for enough to cover the expenses he would incur in entering them in a sale, and he was probably right.

Their pedigrees weren't much, but it wasn't their fault.

"Give them away," I suggested. "It's cheaper than paying me to kill them."

"No," he countered. "If one of them should up and produce a good race horse after I gave them away, I'd never forgive myself."

"But you can 'forgive' yourself for killing five perfectly healthy horses?"

We argued back and forth, and then I suggested he give them away but return their registration certificates to the Jockey Club. Without the registration certificates, any subsequent foals could not be registered, therefore could not be raced.

He didn't think this was a good idea, either. The argument became a shouting match, and I bellowed that I was not going to kill five perfectly healthy animals. He roared back that they were his horses and I was his vet and I'd damn well do what he told me to do.

At that point I screamed back that I was *not* his [bad word] vet anymore, and he knew what he could do with all his horses and his farm and his machinery, too.

He then suggested, rather adamantly, that I get my [rear end] off his [very bad word] property and never show my [same very bad word] face on it again.

Fortunately this all occurred early in the month, and he had already paid his previous month's bill. As it was, he owed me $130, but I guess his check was lost in the mail. It's been more than ten years now.

❧

Another time, a well-educated, seemingly intelligent woman, whom I liked very much and had a great deal of respect for, told me she was no longer able to keep both of her horses. I have very few pleasure horse clients, and she was one.

She lived in an apartment in town but owned two pleasure/show horses, which she boarded at a farm that boarded only this type of horse. There were nearly fifty animals on this place, representing probably forty different owners, each of whom chose his/her own vet. As a result, there were at least a dozen of us coming and going there all the time. To say that this farm actually "boarded" these animals is to use the word in its loosest sense; paddocks, stalls and water were provided, but the owners were responsible for everything else—hay, grain, straw, work, etc.

The rates charged by this farm were not cheap, and an increase had been announced, hence this woman's decision to cut her horse holdings by 50 percent.

"Which one will go?" I asked.

"I think Mirabelle. She's older than Chauncy and not nearly as pretty."

Mirabelle was a nine- or ten-year-old Quarter Horse with an unusually good disposition, but she was mousy brown and sort of dumpy. Chauncy was a bright chestnut Thoroughbred-cross and very racy looking.

"That's probably a good choice," I said. "Mirabelle should make someone a nice riding horse."

"Oh, no!" she exclaimed. "I want you to put her down."

"Put her down! Why, for heaven's sake?"

"No one will take care of her like I do. I couldn't bear to see her treated poorly. And besides, she'd miss me too much."

An exchange similar to the one with the earlier owner ensued, although we kept it on a less profane level, but the result was the same: I ended up with one fewer client. This one didn't owe me anything, however.

❧

As I have related earlier, Stanislas Craft would send me the mares he was going to breed to Kentucky stallions. The quality of Stan's stock was outstanding, and he usually bred to stallions in the $25,000 to $50,000 range and sometimes up to $100,000. In the particular year we are talking about, I had six of his mares, including one named Always Angie.

This was the third breeding season in a row Angie had been with me. Stan always sent pedigrees with the mares the first year they came so I could keep accurate records. Angie's pedigree had preceded her the first year she came down from New York.

What a pedigree it was! Although she herself was unraced, she was a full sister to a Horse of the Year in Europe and to a top stakes winner in England, and a half-sister to an American champion and to three other U.S. stakes winners. Her dam had been a top-notch English stakes winner, and her sire had been champion twice in this country and at the time was the world's leading Thoroughbred sire. It was one of the finest pedigrees I had ever seen.

And with a pedigree like that, I was anxious to see Angie. She was four years old that first year and that would be her first year being bred.

About a week after I received the pedigree, the van bringing Angie and three other of Stan's mares arrived.

The average Thoroughbred is a large animal, usually around sixteen hands and weighing 1,100 or 1,200 pounds. (A "hand" is four inches, and the height of a horse is measured from the ground to the top of the withers; a sixteen-hand horse is, therefore, five feet, four inches tall. The range of size that will probably take in 90 to 95 percent of the adult Thoroughbred population is 15.1 to 16.3 hands, although both extremes are uncommon. Weight range is usually 900 to 1,400 pounds.)

"Wait'll you see what we brought you, Doc," said Jim, the van driver who frequently brought New York horses to me. "You ain't gonna believe it!"

He opened the van, and he and his attendant each led a mare off and I began to walk into the van to get one of the remaining two.

"You get the one there on the left, Doc." He was grinning.

I stepped into the van and turned to the one he had indicated.

"Jim," I called. "You're kidding!"

"No, I ain't, Doc. That's one of Mr. Craft's mares."

There in front of me was a little bitty chestnut mare, maybe 14.2 hands and not weighing more than 700 pounds.

Thoroughbreds have been described as having the "Look of Eagles." It's a great description; I have seen it in the eyes of many, many horses over the years. This little mare, though, could best be described as having the "Look of Opossums." There was no sharp, eager, intelligent glint in these eyes; they were just like two soft, brown mudholes.

Thoroughbreds are alert, especially ones in strange surroundings. They flare their nostrils for strange smells, they prick their ears for strange sounds. They're so intent on seeing strange sights that they often jump from shadows. The two mares that Jim and his helper held were tense and alert, and the one in the van across the aisle from me was pawing the floor of the van and snorting, letting me know that she wanted out of there.

This one, though, just stood there. Her ears may have been pricked, but no one could tell. Normally a horse's ears stand straight up from the top of the head; these didn't. The term "lop-eared" described her: The ears sort of come out from the sides of the head. The look lends the animal neither an alert nor an intelligent appearance.

"Goodness, Jim, who is this?" I asked.

"I don't know, Doc. Check her halter."

Most halters have a brass nameplate on the strap on the left side of the face. A lot of reasons are given for this, but the main one is so the people working with horses can tell them apart. This is a poor reflection on the observation abilities of these folks; no two horses look alike any more than any two people look alike.

(Actually, there may be a problem there, too. I don't know about other people in other fields of endeavor in other parts of the country, but with horse people in horse country there is an increasingly popular item of attire among members of both sexes—a leather belt with a brass nameplate over the left hip. I can see where this can be of immense value. Say you're at a party. You see a person you have met before but can't remember the person's name. Two possible names come to mind, so you sneak a peek at the person's left hip, and lo and behold, it's Bart Thompson, not Susie Billings.)

I looked at the halter. I was stunned by what I read. There, engraved in plain block letters on the brass nameplate, was "Always Angie." Always Angie! The pedigree of the century belonged to this . . . this . . . pony! This lop-eared, dead-headed, doe-eyed pony!

When I was younger and unmarried, I drew a lot of criticism because I placed great value on aesthetics. I would not date someone unless she was good-looking. Actually, I preferred beautiful. In those days I found that I didn't even want to be friends with women who weren't knockouts. (Thankfully, in time I matured and have gone on to have many women friends who would never be centerfolds. And, fortunately, in my younger days, the women I dated did not have the same criteria as I did.)

I would not have dated Angie. We wouldn't even have been friends. Angie was not just unattractive, she was ugly.

I learned to be very fond of her in time, though. She was maybe the most agreeable mare I have ever worked with. When she saw you coming she'd meet you at the gate. She walked onto vans with no fuss and rode quietly. She'd stand calmly to be palpated or specked.

One day in Angie's second year with us, my assistant, Laurie, had a dentist appointment and left at noon. We had both forgotten we needed to palp Angie so we could book her. My wife was shopping and wouldn't be home until too late (the booking office closed at four-thirty) and the kids had after-school activities, so I was there alone.

Angie and her foal came to me as soon as I entered their pad-dock. I snapped a shank on Angie's halter and walked down her right side, talking quietly to her and holding the shank in my right hand. When I reached her hip, I slid my sleeved and lubed arm under her tail and slowly into her rectum. She responded by putting her head down and taking a bite of clover! (This is *not* a recommended method of palpation.)

I know: We began this discussing euthanasia and now we seem to be far afield. Be patient.

Angie got in foal each year I had her. The third year, though, the result of the second year's mating was twins.

Twins are very undesirable in horses for several reasons. First, the uterus of the mare is not made for multiple conceptions. Cows can have twins, sheep can have triplets and even quadruplets, dogs can have litters of ten or twelve or more, a certain little critter called the multimammate mouse can have up to twenty-eight-lets; their uteri are so designed. But the mare is designed for but one, and the usual result of a twin conception is either a spontaneous abortion somewhere along the way or, if the pregnancy goes to term, one or both foals being weak or sickly and dying.

Occasionally a mare carries twins full term and both are viable, and this leads to reason two: The live twin or twins, for reasons that escape me, do not perform as well athletically as single-birth foals, so the owner does not have as much racing potential, resulting in an increased chance that he will offer the twin(s) for sale in one of the many Thoroughbred auctions around the country. Thus, reason three. Twins must be registered as such, thereby being catalogued as such in a sale. Buyers don't want to buy a twin because of the decreased ability to perform, and they don't want a filly twin as a potential broodmare because, as in people, twinning tends to run in families.

There is a clause in most stallion contracts whereby the mare owner is protected. If the mare does not have a live foal that can stand and nurse, no stud fee is payable. Also, in many contracts, if the mare produces twins, neither of which is registered, no stud fee is due.

The sire of Angie's twins was Laughing Flyer, the champion two-year-old of his year. His stud fee was listed as "private," which means if you have to ask, you can't afford it. Stan told me he signed a $40,000 contract with the stipulations mentioned above. Laughing Flyer's first crop had passed through the sales ring the previous year, and each had averaged about $200,000. A foal by him out of Angie would have been worth at least that, if Stan chose to sell it. A twin would be lucky—really lucky—to bring the stud fee.

One of Angie's twins was very small, about the size of a Cocker Spaniel, and unable to stand or, indeed, even roll up on his chest. He died within thirty minutes of birth.

The other, also a colt, was fairly normal in his actions but also pretty small, with ears just like Angie's. I called Stan the next morning (they were born at one A.M.) and broke the news to him.

"Grant, I can't pay a $40,000 stud fee for what you describe. I think it will be best if you put him down."

"There's no reason to put him down, Stan," I protested. "Just don't register him. There'll be no money to pay that way."

"Look, it's the end of May. Angie will be coming home in a few weeks, and I'll have a useless foal up here. Most of them turn out that way, anyhow, but I don't need one that I already *know* won't be worth a hoot. No, put him down and send a certificate to the stud farm so they won't send me a bill."

I almost argued, but I knew it wouldn't do any good. I told him I'd take care of it, even though I had no intention of putting the colt down. I sent a veterinary certificate to the stud farm stating that Always Angie had foaled dead twins, but now I had to figure out what to do with her foal. He would not be euthanized.

We had some friends from church, Ron and Vanetta Willis, who had two daughters, Ronni and SueAnn, who were horse crazy. They would frequently bring the girls to our place where they could visit the horses. They really liked Angie because she wasn't too big and because she was so agreeable.

The Willises' home was on four acres, not a farm but large enough for a horse. I called Ron.

"You want a horse for the girls?" I asked.

"We've talked about it for years, but we just can't afford to buy one," he replied.

"How about a free one?" I told him about the colt.

He said he'd present the idea to the family and call me back. About thirty seconds later the phone rang. It had evidently been a short presentation.

"Everyone says we want him," Ron said. "The girls want to come see him right now. Can we come out?"

At this point, of course, they couldn't take him. He'd have to grow a little and then be weaned. The little guy was not even twenty-four hours old, but he was a very quiet foal. He didn't hide behind his mom or run from people or, worse, try to kick. He walked right up to anyone and allowed himself to be petted and rubbed, truly his mother's child. I told him to bring them on.

It was May 23. Angie would leave sometime in early July. Weaning at six weeks is not easily done, and Angie would still have a full udder. Stan would know she had had a foal on her. Obviously, I had not thought this plan out thoroughly.

We skipped Angie's foal heat but gave her the hormone injection that would cause her to come back in season sooner than she normally would. It was late in the breeding season, and we needed to gain a little time. On June 10 she was ready to be bred, so I booked her and arranged for a van to take her to the breeding shed.

When a mare is sent to be bred, the foal stays behind in a stall. This is often met with serious disapproval from both parties. The mare, when she realizes her foal is not with her, will frequently not willingly enter the van and will whinny frantically for the foal. Once loaded onto the van, she will rear up and/or kick the walls and continue to holler.

Meanwhile, her foal, closed alone in a stall, will scream and buck and fling itself against the walls or door. This usually goes on until the van drives away and the two are out of earshot. Then they generally quiet down, although both still remain nervous and unhappy.

But this didn't happen with Angie and her foal. She walked calmly onto the van and stood quietly as she was closed in. Her foal watched her for a moment through the stall door, then went over to a corner and nibbled on a little hay.

And, typically, when the mare comes back she is anxious to get back to her foal and the foal will rush to her to get the security of the nipple. But not these two. After being away for more than an hour, Angie walked leisurely back to her stall, and the foal, still nibbling on the hay, looked over at her when Laurie put her in, nickered what was probably "Hi, Mom," and took another bite of hay before he walked over to her.

We expected something like this. It had been almost the same way the previous year, although that foal had been a little happier to see her return.

Out in the field, the foal would roam far and wide. Some foals won't go ten feet from their dams; some mares won't let their foals stray. Angie and the foal were in a paddock with three other mares with foals about the same age. Angie's was the youngest, but the oldest was only about three weeks older. It was not unusual to see Angie's colt at the other end of the paddock from her, playing with another foal or sniffing at another mare.

Now it was getting closer to crunch time. Within a month, Stan's mares and foals would be leaving and he was expecting a foal-less, nonlactating Angie.

But then the Fates smiled. Nike Queen, an older mare also owned by Stan, colicked on June 20. Bad colic—she had to have surgery. Nike Queen's foal was four months old, so we weaned him when his mom had to be hospitalized.

The stress of surgery and the removal of the foal will usually cause a mare's milk to dry up, but Queenie was a *very* heavy milker. When she came back to the farm on June 24, she still had a decent bag. Her foal was doing very well without her, but still I was tempted to put them back together.

Queenie was a good-natured mare, not as docile as Angie but still very agreeable. Laurie knew I was concerned about Angie and her foal and how she was going to go back to Stan.

"Why don't you put Angie's foal on Queen?" she suggested.

"She'd never take him, and besides, she has to leave, too."

"Can't she stay a little longer to recover from the surgery?"

Maybe she could. It was worth a try.

We put Queenie in a paddock with only Angie and the colt. After a few minutes of watching each other, the two mares went about their own business. In a little while, the colt walked over to see who this newcomer was. He was a month old and very curious. Queenie just stood there and did nothing.

"Laurie," I said, "grab Angie and take her over to the tobacco barn." The horse barn is what we normally use, and the tobacco barn is on the other side of the farm. I had built four stalls in it, and we used it only when the horse population was too great for the horse barn to hold them all.

We both went in the field, and the foal came to greet us. I held him by his halter while Laurie walked on over to Angie, snapped the shank to her halter and led her toward the gate. As they passed through the gate, Angie looked back at her colt and let out a short whinny. The colt nickered once in reply and Laurie continued to lead Angie off to the tobacco barn.

I turned the little guy loose. He glanced toward his disappearing dam for a moment, then walked over to the waterer and took a drink.

Laurie put Angie in a stall and came back to the field. I stayed for another ten minutes or so, but then I had to leave.

"Just stay here and watch these two," I told her. "Obviously, try not to let the foal get hurt." I'm not sure how she would have prevented it, but I had to say it.

I made a couple of vet calls and got back home in about two hours. Laurie was still standing at the fence, watching Queenie and Angie's foal.

"Any problems?" I asked.

"No," she replied, "and there won't be. He nursed her! About half an hour after you left he went over to her and began sniffing around her belly. He must have touched her bag because she squealed and picked up a leg like she might kick. It scared me to death!

"But then he reached up under her and was obviously nursing. And he did it again just a few minutes ago."

"What about Angie? Has she fussed?"

"I haven't heard a peep out of her."

It all worked out great. Queenie's foal was weaned, Queenie adopted Angie's foal, and Angie's bag dried up. I called Stan and told him an out-and-out lie; I said Queenie needed to stay a few extra weeks to fully recover from her surgery. He thought it was a good idea.

On July 6 Angie, Queenie's foal and the rest of Stan's mares and foals shipped out to New York. Queenie and Angie's foal stayed behind. He was about seven weeks old, and I figured in three to five more weeks we could successfully wean him and send Queenie on home, too (after a few days to allow her to dry up).

The foal had been named by this time. Ronni and SueAnn had decided to call him Sir Prancelot, Prancie for short. Prancie did well and grew well, and on July 31 we decided to wean him. It, too, was uneventful and on August 10 we loaded a dried-up Queenie on a northbound van. Through lies and deceit, she had stayed with us over a month more than she had to, but I never billed Stan for that time. He asked about it once and I told him I'd do it, but I never did.

We hauled Prancie over to the Willises' place in mid-August, where he was treated like visiting royalty. At two he was broken and at three he was shown a little. He's approaching middle age now, and the girls have gone on to other things. Ronni is out of college and working in a city several hundred miles away and SueAnn is in college, also several hundred miles away. Prancie is not wanting for company, however; Ron probably likes him more than his daughters ever did and spends all the time he can with him and riding him.

There is a postscript on Angie. Stan sent her back again the next year and she foaled an unimpressive filly. She was bred back, and Stan sold her at the annual breeding stock sale that November, where she brought only $37,000. Her pedigree was worth a million, but her looks weren't worth a plugged nickel; the $37,000 was evidently a compromise.

That last filly she had for Stan went on to race well, placing in a few stakes and earning nearly $100,000. Then the foal she was carrying when she was sold, also a filly, did the same—placed in several stakes and earned just over $100,000. Her first foal had run in only one race before an injury ended his career.

❦

Maybe five years after Angie was sold, a new client came to me and asked me to check out a few mares he was considering buying privately. We drove to a big-name local farm and they brought out, one at a time, four mares for us to see.

My client was a wealthy man, and these were expensive mares. As each was brought out, he told me their names, a few highlights of their pedigrees, and the asking price. The first one was $200,000, the second $300,000, the third $150,000.

Then came the fourth.

"This is the one I *really* want," he said. "Her name is Always Angie, and her pedigree is one of the finest I've ever seen. They want $400,000 for her."

"Always Angie? I know her," I said.

The groom brought out a beautiful, sixteen-hand, bright chestnut mare. A heavy-bodied, big-boned mare, she must have weighed 1,300 pounds. Alertly pricked atop her head were two attentive ears; nostrils were flared and eyes were wide as she pranced out in front of strangers.

These wide eyes were bright and eager. Maybe they didn't have the Look of Eagles, but they sure had the Look of Pretty Hungry Hawks.

Long ago and far away, if she had been a woman, I would have dated her. Or tried to. This was centerfold on the hoof.

"Isn't she beautiful?" said my client with a sigh.

"She sure is," I agreed, "but this is the wrong mare."

"No, that's her," he assured me. "They showed her to me when I was out here yesterday."

I looked at her halter. Sure enough, there it was: a shiny brass nameplate with "Always Angie" engraved on it.

This was back in the days before Thoroughbreds were blood-typed for identification purposes. In those days, many underhanded things were done in the business. If a top mare's foal died or was a poor individual, an unscrupulous horseman would substitute a foal from a lesser mare and register it as the good mare's foal. An unsuspecting buyer would spend a lot of money for a good pedigree, and when it turned out not to be able to race successfully, it was just written off as the luck of the draw.

What I imagine happened to Angie is this: Someone found a good-looking chestnut mare with similar white markings and put her off as Angie with Angie's registration papers, then sold her to some trusting soul. I hate to think what the real Angie's fate was, but I suspect it involved dog food.

I took my client aside and told him that this mare was *not* Always Angie. I thought he believed me because we left the farm then, but later I learned he went back two days later with another vet and bought her as well as the $200,000 mare. He also never called me again, so I guess euthanasia ended up costing me another client.

Out of curiosity, I checked to see what Angie, or the mare identified as Angie, had produced after her second stakes-placed runner. Neither of her two subsequent foals that had reached racing age had won even one race. This proved nothing, but I suspected the change was made after her new owner got the foal she was carrying at the time Stan sold her. A few years later, I thought of Angie again when we were visiting the Willises, so when we got home I looked up her produce record. Only one of the six foals she produced after Stan had sold her had been a winner, and that one had won only a single race. The stallions she had been bred to looked like a Who's Who of horsedom, so she had every chance.

Since the advent of blood-typing, cheating such as this has been drastically reduced.

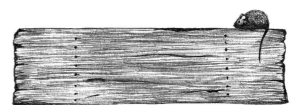

HOLLYWOOD II: THE SEQUEL

Over the years since the making of *The Thoroughbred*, I have had a few other contacts with Hollywood personalities.

I don't like parties. I can think of dozens of better things to do than dress uncomfortably and go somewhere and stand around all evening in the middle of a bunch of strangers.

My wife, though, does not share my feelings. She likes parties.

And well she should. She doesn't view the necessary attire as uncomfortable. Quite the contrary; she *enjoys* wearing clothes you couldn't clean stalls in. And she doesn't look upon the other party-goers as strangers; by the end of an evening she will have met most of them and made friends with several.

That's just one of our many differences. Years ago I saw a little poem credited to Anonymous that went something like this:

She is a creature of the night,
By nine I'm safe in bed.
Why did we wait to find this out
'Til after we were wed?

That is pretty applicable to most aspects of our relationship.

By way of compromise, we go to *some* parties. Not all, mind you, just enough to make me dread little square envelopes in the mail.

There was another horse racing movie made around here. I don't remember the name or the plot, but it, too, centered on a horse and the daughter of a farm owner. To the best of my knowledge, it was never released.

The only performer in it anyone had ever heard of was Jacques Patton, who played the farm owner. I guess at some point in his career he had had large parts in movies, but I had only seen him in TV shows where he was usually billed as "Special Guest Star." He was either killed off early or he was the bad guy. Sometimes a little of each.

I was not a "technical adviser" on this movie, so I never really met any of the cast. But there was a party given at a local country club just before filming began, and at this party the cast was introduced. For reasons unclear to me we received an invitation, and my wife wanted to go. We went.

About an hour after the supposed starting time of the party, a big shot in the local horse industry popped up with a microphone and asked for our attention, which we gave him. He asked us to gather 'round; the cast was to be introduced now.

First, two men I'd never heard of or seen before were named, and they came forward together, smiling and waving. They were short.

Next came a young man, Tom something, and a young woman. They were short, too. Then a little girl was introduced by herself. She looked to be seven or eight, but because of the sizes of everyone else she was probably fifteen. A middle-aged woman was introduced next; this was probably the "mother." And finally, Jacques Patton, the star, was introduced. He was maybe five-five. I was now convinced that there was a cutoff height for actors and actresses.

(This may sound as if I have a problem with short people. I don't. In fact, I like a lot of them. My wife is maybe five-three, if you don't flatten her hair when you measure her.)

The cast proceeded to mingle. Ol' Jacques walked up to me, shook my hand, said, "I'm happy to meet you," and immediately went on to someone else before I had a chance to say anything. I'm not sure that really constitutes "meeting" someone.

A few minutes later Tom something came by and shook my hand, too, and then moved on just as quickly. I asked Barb if we could leave. We couldn't, so I spent the evening eating little turkey sandwiches. I love turkey sandwiches, so it wasn't a total loss.

It wasn't 'til a couple of years later that the next celebrity contact came. We were invited to a party given by a major consignor to the summer yearling sales. He gave a party every year, but until now our invitation had always seemed to get lost in the mail, and the last thing I expected this year was one. A few months before, I had been called upon to testify in a court case involving him, and my testimony was for the other guy. The other guy won. Maybe he intended to poison my punch.

This annual bash was a big social event. The thrower of the party always had a celebrity "guest" in attendance, and rumor had it that his "guest" usually cost him around $50,000 to "invite." This year's guest was to be the world-famous comedian Don House. House had been in show business for half a century and had appeared in dozens of movies, made countless TV specials, and journeyed all over the world entertaining our troops. He was a legend.

We went to the party, of course; Barb's will prevailed. House was there, being led around by two young ladies who evidently weren't paid very much because they couldn't afford full outfits. The seamstress must have started at the bottom, then apparently run out of material just as she was getting to the upper extremes of the gowns. The poor young women were just *barely* covered in these areas. It's a good thing it was a warm evening; with their physiques, a chest cold could have been disastrous.

These girls were never going to make it in Hollywood, though. They were both tall, maybe five-ten or -eleven. Previous experience told me that five-ten or -eleven was just too tall. Don House was a much more Hollywoodish five-eight or so.

The evening consisted of this little old man (House) wandering among the guests saying things that, if you or I said them, would have gotten us busted in the mouth. The most interesting aspect of all this was the fact that most of the guests actually *laughed* when he insulted them.

I began to give strong consideration to throwing away any mail in the future that even remotely resembled an invitation.

The next year I had what was to be my best experience with celebrities. It was early May, and the breeding season was in full swing. I came home one evening late—nine or ten—and there was a message for me to call Ronald Porter. The number had a 703 area code, which was northern Virginia.

Years before, when I was fresh out of school, I had done a little vet work for a Ronald Porter. He was some sort of government employee in Washington who owned a small farm and a couple of broodmares in the Virginia countryside where I was employed. I hadn't heard anything from or about him since we moved to Kentucky, so I wasn't sure this was the same guy.

The message said to call whenever I got in, so at around ten I dialed the number.

A woman answered, and I told her I was returning Ronald Porter's call.

"Just a moment," she said, and evidently handed the phone to someone. I heard her say, "Grant Kendall for you."

The next voice was a man's. "Grant! Thanks for calling. This is Ron Porter. Do you remember me?"

I said, "Of course. How are you?"

We exchanged the usual small talk, then he said, "Grant, I need a favor. Some friends of mine have just gotten into the horse business, and they have two mares boarded down there in Lexington. They're going to be in Louisville for the Derby on Saturday and want to come over to Lexington on Sunday to see their mares and the stallions they're being bred to. Can you show them around?"

Oh me, I thought. "Golly, Ron, things are pretty busy. If it doesn't take too long, I can try."

We talked on. It turned out his friends were Mandy Brandon and her husband, Nick Willets. I had never heard of him, but Ron said he was a movie director and just happened to be his nephew or cousin or something.

Mandy was a different story, however. She was famous and had won the Oscar for best actress the previous year. I hadn't seen her Academy Award–winning movie, but then I haven't seen an award-winning movie for years.

But I had seen Mandy in one movie. She was acclaimed as a great actress, but in all honesty I couldn't see much difference between her performance and that of 90 percent of the other actresses I'd seen. The most discernible difference between Mandy and the others was her looks. She was attractive, certainly, but not beautiful. I'd much rather pay my money to see beautiful than I would to see attractive, but as well as I can figure, this is why her performances were acclaimed. I mean, look at the actresses over the years who have been lauded for their talent—overall, not a group of knockouts. Give me Marjorie Fallon any day.

So much for editorializing. Mandy and Nick, Ron told me, loved horses and horse racing, so they had bought a farm in Virginia and stocked it with two broodmares for starters. They weren't great mares, but they were certainly in the upper end of the spectrum. They purchased them at the November auction the previous year, one for $102,000 and the other for $75,000.

While at the sale, they had met Wallace Arnholm, general manager of Mailesmere Farm and owner of Arnholm Farm. Recognizing a potentially important source of new money in the horse business, Arnholm proceeded to sell them breeding seasons in two of the stallions standing at Mailesmere, and he also convinced them to board their two mares at his own farm while they were in Kentucky to be bred. Why arrangements weren't made through him to show the Willetses around, I don't know.

I agreed to be their host for a few hours, and a time and place were set for me to meet them Sunday morning, the day after the Derby, at an easy-to-find location just off the interstate north of Lexington. I called the number listed for Arnholm Farm, and when the woman who answered told me that Mr. Arnholm did not live on the farm, I told her that a couple of owners would be stopping by to see their mares. I gave her the Willetses' name, and she said, "Yeah, I think I know them mares." It wasn't necessary to call Mailesmere Farm because the breeding season was in full force and there would be mares and people coming and going there all day long anyhow.

I arrived at the meeting location about five minutes early. A tall young man perhaps in his early thirties was standing there. "Are you Grant Kendall?" he asked. I said I was, and he introduced himself. "Nick Willets. We really appreciate you doing this." Then he suggested we go in their car. "I think we'll have more room," he said.

We sure did. Somehow—our taxes at work, no doubt—they had acquired the use of a state-owned limousine, complete with driver, who happened to be a plainclothes state policeman. I sat in front with the cop, a pleasant individual who contributed very little to the conversation.

Mandy, in the back with Nick, looked exactly as she did on the screen. They had attended a party the previous evening in Louisville and she admitted to being exhausted, but Nick had either gone to bed early or weathered the festivities well because he was in peak form. Mandy asked, if the need arose, to be introduced as Mandy Willets.

I directed the driver to Arnholm Farm. I knew where it was, but I'd never been there. The first thing we noticed when we turned in was the fence; it was in dire need of a fresh coat of paint. And as we headed up the driveway to the barn, it appeared as if the guy who did the painting may well have been the mower, too. The grass was nearly a foot tall, and weeds were thriving. Thistles four feet tall dotted the paddocks.

When we arrived at the barn, we couldn't find anyone. (The barn had apparently been painted at the same time as the fences.) I called out for someone, but there was no answer. I checked the time; we were there within ten minutes of when I said we'd be.

There were no horses in the stalls, but in a large field behind the barn we found several mares and foals. "Are your mares foaling mares?" I asked.

They were, so I asked their names and went in the field to see if I could find them. Nick recognized one, which was a good thing because her halter had no nameplate on it. Eventually we found the other one, too.

They were dirty and ungroomed, and their feet—foals' as well as mares'—badly needed to be trimmed. Mandy, who had remained outside the field and walked around the area to look around, came back and said to Nick, "There are planks over there falling off the posts. How much are we paying to board here?"

(Before we proceed, let me say this: I had not seen Mandy stand up until we got out of the limousine at Arnholm Farm. She was a normal-size, almost tall woman, probably five-eight. My theory of a size limit was being tested.)

"Twenty-five dollars a day per mare," Nick replied. Then he said to me, "Are we being screwed?"

I didn't know what to say. The ethics of the horse industry are low; it's the rule rather than the exception to knock the other guy at every opportunity, but as a vet I couldn't do that. I began, "Well, this *is* the busiest time of the whole year and they've probably gotten a little behind . . ." but before I got any further, a pickup drove up to the barn and a very large, very heavy man struggled out of it.

"What you doin' there?" he demanded.

I answered. "I called a couple of days ago. These are the Willetses; they're here to see their horses."

"Oh, yeah. My wife said sumpin' 'bout it. Which'uns are yourn?" He spat a gob of tobacco juice, which left a brown line of drool down his chin. He wiped it off with the back of his hand, looked at the hand, then wiped it off on his shirt. From the looks of the shirt, this was a common occurrence.

"Who takes care of the horses here?" Mandy asked.

"Why, I do! I'm the manager of this here farm!" He beamed, showing a few brown teeth and several spaces where teeth had formerly resided.

"Who helps you?" she continued.

"There's jest me! I do it all." He looked at her closely. "Say, ain't I seen you somewheres? Ain't you been out here before?"

"No. Doesn't Mr. Arnholm manage his own farm?"

"Shoot, no! He ain't got the time. He's allus over to Mailesmere. Besides, he got me here."

Nick spoke. "What's the status of our mares?"

"Status? What's that?"

"Are they back in foal or what?"

"Which'uns are yourn?"

"Society Flame and Garden Spot."

"Oh, them. Lessee, ol' Flame's been stuck, I 'member that. Garden Spot—yep, I think she's been stuck, too."

"Stuck?" questioned Mandy.

"Bred," I explained.

"Then they're in foal?" Nick continued.

"Yeah, I think they might be. See, my wife, she writes all this stuff down and she ain't here right now. Mr. Arnholm, he sends you a bill and it's got all that stuff on it, don't it?"

As we were leaving, Mandy said, "Grant, where can we send our mares? They can't stay here."

Oh my, I thought. I can't tell her where to send their mares. If Arnholm found out, all hell would break loose.

"The breeding season's nearly over," I said. "Why don't you just leave them here and then send them someplace else next year?"

"Do you own any mares?" she asked.

"Yeah, two."

"Where do you keep them?"

"At home. We have a small farm."

"Do you keep mares for other people?"

Oh, no. She was going to ask if I would take their mares. Within a week the word would be all over central Kentucky that a vet—me—was stealing boarders, the most prized commodities in the whole breeding industry.

"Oh, a few, I guess." I tried to act nonchalant. "But I don't actively search out boarders."

"May we see your place?" asked Nick.

"Uhhhh," I began. "Sure. But Arnholm . . ."

"Isn't taking proper care of our horses," Mandy interrupted.

"There's the matter of ethics."

"You haven't done anything unethical," she said.

"That's not how Arnholm will see it. And that's not what will be spread around the countryside. As a vet, I have to be pretty careful."

"May we see your farm?" Nick asked again.

I directed our driver. Now to say that the grass was always neatly mowed and the weeds properly eaten would be stretching it a bit, but it happened that the previous week Laurie's boyfriend had been out of work (not an unusual scenario for him), so I had hired him to mow and trim. As a result, the place was looking pretty good. Nick and Mandy liked it. (In my defense, even when behind on mowing we don't have four-foot-tall thistles.)

Even though they said they liked it, they didn't say anything else about moving their mares, and I certainly didn't bring it up.

I directed the driver to Mailesmere Farm, where the stallions stood that their mares were being bred to and where Wallace Arnholm held forth as general manager. It was a little after eleven A.M. I knew the morning breedings would still be going on, so I had the driver take us to the breeding shed. There were still four or five mares waiting to be bred.

Mailesmere Farm was the other end of the spectrum from Arnholm Farm. The miles and miles of fencing were repainted annually, the entire farm—some 450 acres—was mowed weekly, there were sixty or seventy people employed to care for about two hundred resident horses. The stallion complex, which consisted of the breeding shed and eight stallion barns, was rumored to have cost $8 million to build. It was an impressive operation.

I was worried about what the Willetses would say to Arnholm if he was there, and what they planned to do with their horses. Just before we got out of the car, Mandy asked, "Grant, will you do the veterinary work on our mares the rest of the season if we leave them with Arnholm?"

This wasn't too bad. I still wasn't crazy about it, and I didn't know whom Arnholm used as a vet. I was sure the presiding vet wouldn't like it. I know I wouldn't if I was in his position (*prima donna* is Latin for "equine vet"), but still, I wasn't taking anyone's boarders.

Before I could answer, she added, "At least we'd feel someone with our interests in mind would be seeing them occasionally."

Now if I was really the altruistic person I like to think I am, I would have told her that any vet who cared for their horses would have their interests in mind. If the mares in our care don't get in foal, several things can happen. If it is a boarded mare, she may well not return to the same farm next year; therefore we lose a mare to work on and, therefore, a mare to charge for. And, even worse, if enough mares don't get in foal, the farm will replace the vet and we lose a whole farm full of mares to charge for. Self-preservation causes us to be *very* concerned over the mares of clients. So much for altruism.

So I agreed to do it. "If it's all right with Arnholm."

"And next year, will you keep them at your place?" Nick asked.

That was certainly all right. A lot of people don't return to the same farm year after year, and it's not likely Arnholm would even know where the Willetses moved them to.

We went into the breeding shed. There was a board on the wall that listed the stallions to be bred that session.

"Which horses did your mares go to?" I asked.

"Northern Rocker and French Reunion," Nick said.

These were two nice young stallions. It was French Reunion's third year at stud, and he had a $25,000 fee. Northern Rocker had just been syndicated into forty shares at $250,000 a share; his fee was $50,000.

The board showed that French Reunion had had a mare that morning so he would be in his stall, but Northern Rocker was not listed. He'd be out in his paddock.

I went to look for the stallion manager, to have him have someone show us around. As I walked away, a young woman who was there with a mare approached Mandy and asked, "Are you Mandy Brandon?" Mandy said she was, and the girl asked for her autograph.

I found Joe Hopper, the stallion manager, and told him what we needed. When I returned to the Willetses with a stud groom, Mandy was still signing autographs.

The groom took us to the adjacent stallion barn and brought out French Reunion, a plain-looking, medium-size dark bay horse. Neither Nick nor Mandy was impressed by him. He was very ordinary.

The groom said, "Rocker's outside. His paddock's a couple hundred yards off. You wanna walk or drive?"

They wanted to walk, and as we exited the barn, a car drove up, honking. Wallace Arnholm hopped out, beaming. "Mandy! Nick! Joe called and said you were here! You should've called me." Then, to me, "Hello, Dr. Kendall. Nice to see you." He said it with as much enthusiasm as he might have said, "My apple has a worm in it."

The Willetses responded coolly. After the initial exchange of moderate pleasantries, Mandy said—she didn't ask—"Dr. Kendall will provide the veterinary care for our mares."

Arnholm said nothing for a moment. He looked from her to me and back to Nick, then smiled broadly. "Of course! That's great! We'll have him out tomorrow to check them!" He turned to me. "Dr. Kendall, please come by in the morning."

Arnholm wanted to know what he could do for the Willetses, and they told him the groom was taking excellent care of them. Arnholm stood and watched as we walked down the lane to Northern Rocker's paddock.

"I don't think he liked that," Nick said.

"I don't care," Mandy answered.

When we reached the paddock, the groom placed a lead shank on Northern Rocker and brought him out to show him off. He was a beautiful horse—far more striking than French Reunion—and he had evidently been groomed earlier that morning. His coat was shining, and every hair was in place in his mane and tail.

"Man, he's gorgeous!" exclaimed Nick.

"He's marvelous!" Mandy agreed. "Look. Even his feet have been polished. He looks like he's been manicured. I wish somebody would take care of me like that."

I smiled. "He's worth ten million dollars. If you were worth that, maybe someone *would* treat you as well."

"I am and they don't," she said simply.

Only one of the Willetses' mares got in foal that year. They sent them to me to board the next year, and they both conceived, but somewhere along the way the Willetses decided they liked Quarter Horses better than Thoroughbreds, sold those mares and their foals, and bought a few Quarter Horses. I never saw or heard from them again, except in the movies.

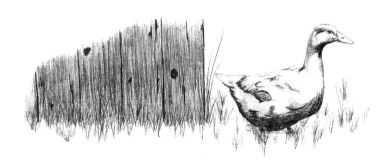

GARY

Earlier I said that a horse will always give a warning before it acts, and that's true. That doesn't mean a horse won't hurt you, because sometimes the time interval between the warning and the action is so short that you can't get to safety soon enough. Also, even though strong warnings are being given, sometimes some things have to be done, so you proceed as carefully as possible. And sometimes, you (not me) go blithely ahead, ignoring the warnings.

Around here, where there may be more horses per capita than anywhere in the world, people are always getting hurt by them. Back about the time I came to Kentucky, a vet was killed by a horse while trying to worm it, and a few years ago an experienced horseman was killed while attempting to help load a mare onto a van.

More recently, I was called to a farm for the first time. When I drove up to the barn, a group of six or seven people were standing around in front of it. I parked and got out of my car, and a man said, "If you're the vet, come see if you can do something for this guy."

The group parted, and I saw a young man lying there on his back on the ground. His eyes were open and he was staring straight up. "I think he's dead," another fellow said.

He sure looked dead. I reached down and felt for his pulse. There wasn't any. "What happened?" I asked.

"We don't know," the first man said. "He was leading a mare out, and the next thing we knew, she ran back into the barn and we found him here."

"When did this happen?"

The men looked at each other. After a moment one of them said, "Oh, maybe ten minutes ago."

"This guy's been lying here for ten minutes and you haven't done anything?"

No one said anything. I went back to the car and dialed 911 on my mobile phone, and within eight or ten minutes an emergency medical vehicle arrived. A few minutes later the helicopter from the university hospital came, and the young man was pronounced dead. Eventually we learned that he had somehow been kicked in the throat, collapsing his trachea so he could not breathe.

I don't know if his life could have been saved if the farm crew had acted more quickly, but I didn't want to work with people who seemed that stupid. I told them they needed to find another vet and left.

Horses are dangerous.

While I have never been killed by a horse, I have been injured. I incurred a minor leg fracture when a mare kicked me. I had a toe broken when one stepped on me. I have been struck in the face by flying front feet twice. I was cow-kicked in the head by a mule. I was cow-kicked in the groin by a colicking mare (for several days I was glad we had children and didn't want any more).

These all hurt, but none stopped me from working. In a couple of cases I limped around for a while, and in a couple of others my vision was reduced for a few days, but life went on. With the exception of the mule kick, all of these were forewarned, but in each case I had to proceed, albeit with great care. Over the years I have worked on hundreds of horses that gave warnings and even reacted, but because of care no one was injured.

Once, though, I was put out of commission.

My old and true clients, Glenraven Farm, have boarded horses off and on for years for Max Dammer, whose farm is in Kansas. It was one of Max's horses that got me.

Max is very wealthy, and one reason he stays that way is because he doesn't fritter away his money on horse care. We assume he has some sort of employee on his Kansas farm, but you couldn't tell it from his animals' behavior. When they arrive in Kentucky, they have *not* been overhandled—i.e., they're as wild as March hares.

A few years ago Max sent ten yearlings to Glenraven, a stopover en route to Aiken, South Carolina, where they were to be broken. These yearlings had been herded onto a cattle trailer in Kansas and then herded off into a barn at Glenraven, where they were chased into stalls.

All horses shipped across a state line are supposed to have negative Coggins tests before shipping, but a whole lot don't, and most of the time vans aren't stopped so the paperwork can be checked. Max's yearlings arrived here without Coggins tests, but they could not ship into the training facility at Aiken without being tested, so Max instructed the Glendons to have me test them while they were here, then ship them on down.

These ten yearlings had been handled, but not enough to do anything but make them afraid of people. On Coggins-taking day, we began at the first stall and went down the line, drawing the necessary blood sample from each horse. We were careful, and although some of them acted pretty nasty, the first nine were bled with no damage to either horses or people.

Number ten, though, was something else entirely. Susan Glendon stepped in the stall to put a shank on him, but before she could get to his head, he reared and struck. He managed to hit both of her arms; nothing was broken but she was out of commission for the day.

There was simply no approaching this colt. He'd strike with his front feet or wheel and kick with his hind feet. Roger Glendon, though, is a cowboy at heart. He lassoed the colt and then snubbed him to a stout corner post in the stall. This did not sit well with the yearling, but it enabled us to (1) get a shank on him, and (2) twitch him.

After applying the twitch and feeling we had the situation under control, Roger released the noose so the colt could breathe. That was a mistake. He began fighting the twitch, but Roger held on. The drawing of the blood would be a matter of but a few seconds and it would be over.

As soon as I stuck the needle through the colt's skin, though, he exploded! To this day, neither Roger nor I know exactly what happened, but somewhere in the melee I was kicked or struck on the outside of my right knee, forcing it to bend inward. This is not a normal knee function. Then, somehow, I was kicked across the stall and ended up lying in a corner.

Roger, meanwhile, was hanging on to the twitch and shank for dear life. He was struck a couple of times, but he held on. The colt was trying to get to me with his hind feet, but Roger kept him directed slightly away.

"Get out!" Roger shouted to me.

Excellent advice, but advice I could not heed. I couldn't get up! My right leg was nonfunctional.

"I can't hold him much longer!" Roger yelled. "Get up and get out!"

I was trying! Finally I crawled out on two hands and one leg, just as the colt reared and pulled both shank and twitch from Roger's hands.

We didn't get the Coggins drawn on the colt that day or for the next ninety days, because that's how long I was out of action. My medial patellar ligament ruptured when the knee was forced inward, and I was in a brace and grounded while it healed. When I did return to work, I still wore the brace for a few more weeks. (There are probably things more painful than this, but I don't want to experience them.)

The doctors told me at my age I may have lingering effects, and I do. The area flares up whenever I stress it, and it will hurt for an hour to a day or more, but basically I'm fully functional. Barb does not totally believe me when I tell her that things such as mowing the lawn and taking out the trash aggravate it and calls me an out-and-out liar when I insist that going to parties causes severe pain.

The title of this chapter is "Gary," and the astute reader will recall that Gary is a socially maladjusted female cat in our household; said reader may also ask, "Are you sure this is the correct chapter?"

Yes.

At the time of my injury, Gary had lived with us for many years; she must have been five years old, anyhow. Many times we would go days without seeing her. She was about three months old when we acquired her, so I don't know what went into making her this way, but as a pet she was useless. I guess she ate and drank, but it was when no one else was around. She used the sandbox, too, because we never found any "accidents." Other than the vaccinations and worming I had given her the day she moved in, she had not received any veterinary care. I assume she stayed healthy, but I didn't know.

Okay, I was hurt. I was in a brace that held my leg straight and I was on painkillers that didn't kill any pain. Spaced me out, yes, but I was spaced out in pain. I was also supposed to be on crutches, but they required a level of coordination I was unable to meet; I was probably safer without them.

Our bedroom is on the second floor. Ascending and descending the stairs was slow and painful, but I managed.

Downstairs, all I could do was sit or lie on the couch and watch TV (daytime TV is indescribably horrid, by the way), but I could *not* get comfortable. I couldn't sit in a normal chair because my leg wouldn't bend, and there was just enough difference in height between the easy chair and the footstool to put a painful angle on my knee. Lying on the couch was only marginally better because the cushions were soft and didn't give enough support.

After the first couple of days of being grounded, in addition to being bored out of my mind, I found my knee would become increasingly painful as the day progressed. By evening it would be extremely painful, whereas in the morning it had only been very painful, so on the third or fourth day I climbed the stairs—slowly— and lay down on the bed for about half an hour. The support the mattress gave helped a lot to ease the discomfort.

That first time I went up, Gary *zoomed* out of the bedroom just as I entered it. Ditto the second day. Apparently she spent her days up there; rarely did anyone go to the second floor before mid-evening, so I guess she looked on it as a secure place to hang out.

After maybe four days of this, Gary's zoom slowed to a scurry. Whether she was getting accustomed to me appearing every day at about the same time—early afternoon—or realized that, with my lack of mobility, I was no threat to her, I don't know. It appeared that she spent her time on the bed, because in her reduced haste to leave, I had seen her jump off the bed as I entered the room.

One day after a couple of weeks of this, she didn't leave the bedroom. She scooted over to a corner of the room and lay there, but kept her eyes on me. This continued for several days, but eventually, instead of eyeing me the whole time I was in the room, she went to sleep.

It was another couple of weeks before the next step. I limped into the room one day and she stayed on the bed. She was obviously very tense and was ready to run if necessary, but she stayed there. I lay down and she very cautiously moved as far from me as she could and still lie on the bed. She remained tense but didn't leave.

"It's okay, Gary," I said, "I'm not going to hurt you." She looked unconvinced.

This went on for several days. One day while I was lying there reading and Gary was on the far side of the bed (I thought), I felt something pushing against my foot. I put my book down and looked to see what it was.

Gary had moved over next to me and was rubbing her head against the side of my foot! I reached for her, slowly, but she moved away. The next day, she rubbed against my leg, but again withdrew when I tried to touch her. This went on every day—foot or leg—and I stopped trying to reach for her.

Then I fell asleep one day. I was awakened by Gary's head rubbing against my hand, and in a few more days she let me rub her in return. I told Barb about it, but I couldn't prove it because Gary ran whenever she came into the room.

But she (Gary, not Barb) and I had become friends. She rubbed against me and I petted her, but only when we were alone together. She became more friendly every day, but when we went to bed for the night she would disappear.

Fang had chosen to spend the nights outside, so we had no bed cat at this point. One night—or I should say one morning—at about three A.M., I felt one of my hands being pushed against. It was Gary asking to be petted. I patted her a couple of times, and then something must have startled her because she jumped down and ran.

I was still pretty immobile and was still being appalled by daytime TV. My seat of choice for this displeasure was the living room couch, which was easily viewed from the stairs to the second floor.

Late one morning, a few days after the middle-of-the-night episode, I was home alone. Our son was off at college and our daughter, now in high school, seemingly only came home to sleep. Barb was shopping, Fang and the dogs were outside, and Annie had been gone two years, having lived to the ripe old age of seventeen, so everything was very quiet when I noticed some movement out of the corner of my eye. I looked over and saw Gary slinking down the stairs. At the bottom she stopped, tensed and looked around, prepared to flee if necessary. When no danger was seen (or imagined), she made two great leaps and landed on the couch.

"Hi, Gary," I said. She stared at me. A minute later she moved next to me and rubbed her head on my hand.

She lay there by me, letting me pet her, for a long time, then the phone rang. She leaped up and tore back up the stairs to the sanctuary of the bedroom, where she stayed until I hobbled up an hour or so later. She lay by my side as I read.

The downstairs visits occurred often from then on, but only when no one else was home. She would also want to be petted most nights. Still, though, no one else was to be trusted.

One night a few weeks later, Barb was having difficulty falling asleep. She was lying there awake but not moving when Gary jumped on the bed. I was asleep, but Barb later told me that Gary began rubbing against my arm and she (Barb) reached over and petted her. Gary sat still for it.

Up to this point in Gary's life, we had only heard one sound from her: a small hiss on the day I brought her home years before. No meows, no purrs, no nothing ever.

The next step in Gary's socialization occurred just before I was able to return to the real world. She had been making nightly bed hops for quite some time and letting Barb touch her (but *not* in the daytime) and had actually appeared downstairs once or twice, albeit hurriedly, when someone other than me was there.

This particular night, Barb and I were awakened by a loud, deep, rumbling noise. Waking me is no great challenge—I'm a very light sleeper—but waking Barb is a trick. I think she goes into a coma every night. But this woke her, too.

And it got louder! And closer!

Then a cat head rubbed against my hand and I realized what it was. Gary was purring!

Apparently years and years of suppressed purrs had finally come to the surface and were being loosed on us. Barb said the bed shook, but it probably didn't.

As time has gone on, the purring has subsided to a fairly normal level, but she still does it only in the middle of the night. Gary comes down more often and will sometimes visit me even if other people are in the room (she will *not* visit them). Too much commotion—a sigh, a weight shift, a leg crossing—will send her zipping off to safety, though.

She's still a long way from normal, but in middle age she has learned a little trust. I'm not sure "love" is what she feels for me, but I think she derives pleasure from my company and I know I enjoy hers. It makes the pain of the kick from Max's yearling worth it, although I don't plan to befriend any more cats in this manner.

I imagine you're saying about now, "Okay, so now you have a tame cat. What happened to the colt?" Well, in the three months I was out of action, the Glendons worked with him—carefully—and he responded as Gary had (without the purr): he liked Susan and he let Roger handle him, but anyone else was still seen as a potential threat.

His buddies had gone on to Aiken, and when I got back to work, we finally got the blood sample for his Coggins test and he joined them. He was broken and trained and raced and I'd like to say he went on to win many races and lots of money for Max, but I can't. He couldn't outrun a rock.

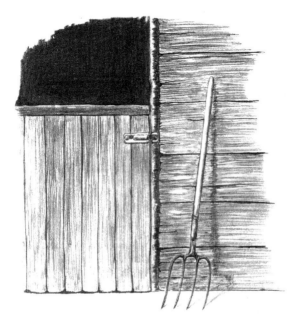

GLOSSARY

AMBULATORY CLINIC A rotation in vet school in which the students make farm calls to treat animals not ill or injured enough to require hospitalization.

ANESTROUS The period of a mare's reproductive cycle during which she is not breedable.

BACKSTRETCH The area of a racetrack where the horses are stabled.

BARREN Describing a mare that was bred but did not conceive.

BAY A horse color, light to dark brown with black mane, tail and lower legs.

BLINKERS Cups or flaps attached to the bridle that prevent a horse from using his peripheral vision and keep him from being distracted.

BLOOD TYPE A method of foal identification and parentage verification.

BOOK (*v.*)   To arrange for the mating of a mare to a stallion.

BREEDING SHED   A building, often attached to a barn, used solely for the mating of mares to stallions.

BROODMARE   A female horse used for foal production.

CANNON   The bone between the knee (front) or hock (rear) and ankle of a horse.

CHESTNUT   A horse color, yellowish to reddish to brown with mane, tail and lower legs of the same color.

CLAIM, CLAIMER OR CLAIMING RACE   A horse for sale in a race; a cheap class of race or horse. A horse entered in a claiming race may be "claimed" by another owner for the claiming price.

COGGINS TEST   A blood test to determine if a horse is positive for equine infectious anemia, a disease spread by biting insects.

COLIC   A sign of abdominal distress; not a specific disease.

COLOSTRUM   "First milk"; necessary for the newborn because it contains important antibodies.

COVER (*v.*)   To breed a mare.

COW KICK   A kick by a hind leg that goes forward or forward and outward; cows can, mules can, most horses can't.

CRADLE   A method to move a horse that doesn't want to move. Two people lock arms across the horse's rear and pull him forward.

CULTURE   A test that shows if there are bacteria present.

DIURETIC   A drug that causes more frequent urination.

DYSTOCIA   Difficult birth.

EAR (*v.*)   To grab a horse's ear and squeeze it in order to control a fractious animal.

EPIPHYSITIS   Inflammation of the growth areas of bones.

ESTROUS CYCLE   The time from one ovulation to the next, typically about three weeks in mares.

EUTHANASIA   Humane destruction.

FARROW (*n.*)   A baby pig; (*v.*) to have a litter of pigs.

FECAL BALLS   Manure. Because of the structure of a horse's intestine, fecal material is usually dropped in small round "balls."

FOAL HEAT   The first heat period a mare has after foaling, usually eight to ten days later.

FOLLICLE   A balloonlike structure that arises on an ovary; it contains the egg.

FOUNDER   An inflammatory condition of the feet of hooved animals.

FURLONG   One-eighth of a mile; used to measure horse races.

GELDING   A male horse that has been castrated.

GROWTH MEDIUM   A mixture of nutrients conducive to bacterial growth.

HIP-LOCK   A birthing complication in which the hips of the neonate become wedged in the birth canal.

HOT WALKER   A person who walks a horse that needs to be cooled out after having been raced or trained.

IN FOAL   Pregnant; a pregnant mare is said to be "in foal."

IN HEAT (in season)   Receptive to the male for breeding.

ISCHIUM   One of the pelvic bones.

JOCKEY CLUB   The governing body, rules-making organ and registration center of the Thoroughbred horse industry.

JOHNSON & JOHNSON   A large manufacturer of medical supplies, especially bandage materials.

JUG   An intravenous solution of vitamins and amino acids given to horses to perk them up or replace deficiencies.

JUMP (*n.*)   To mount a mare by a teaser to see if she will hold still to be bred.

LAMB'S NIPPLE   A rubberized nipple that fits over a bottle end; used for feeding milk to young animals.

LAY-UP (*n.*)   A horse brought from the racetrack to the farm for a period of time to recover from illness or injury.

LEG STRAP   A leather strap, often a belt, used to hold a horse's front leg off the ground in a flexed position so she will not kick. A leg strap is used on mares at breeding.

LET-DOWN (*n.*)   The transition period for horses between the rigors of training and the relative ease of farm life.

LIGHTS   Artificially lengthening the amount of daylight by putting mares in lighted stalls; it causes the mares to begin cycling earlier.

LUBE (*n.*)   A viscous, water-soluble material used primarily to make rectal palpation safer and easier.

MAIDEN   A horse (of either sex) that has not won a race; or a mare that has never been bred.

MASTITIS   Inflammation of the udder.

NASOGASTRIC TUBE   A long, flexible tube that is passed through a nostril, down the esophagus and into the stomach and used to administer certain medications.

ON THE BOARD   Finishing first, second, third or fourth in a horse race; the first four finishers are listed on the tote board.

OSSELET   An inflammation of some of the ankle bones in a horse.

OVULATION   The release of the egg from the follicle.

PALPATE OR PALP   To reach in rectally and feel the internal organs, specifically the ovaries and uterus, in a reproductive exam.

PALPEBRAL REFLEX   The automatic response of the eyelids when the eyeball itself is touched; does not occur after death.

PARASITE OVA   Worm eggs.

PROGESTERONE   A hormone necessary for the maintenance of pregnancy.

PUBIS   One of the pelvic bones.

PULMONARY HEMORRHAGE   Bleeding from the lungs.

RADIOGRAPH   An X ray.

REGISTRATION CERTIFICATE   Proof that a Thoroughbred has been recorded with the Jockey Club; necessary for racing or breeding.

SHANK   A strap, leather or rope, used for leading a horse.

SHEDROW   In a training barn, the area under the overhang where the horses are walked.

SHOW (*v.*)   Respond positively to a teaser.

SLIP (*v.*)   Abort.

SPAY   To remove the reproductive organs of a female animal.

SPEC/SPECKING (*v.*)   To examine using a speculum.

SPECULUM   A tube used to visualize the vagina and cervix.

STAKE (*n.*)   The highest class of horse race.

STALLION SEASON   The right to breed a mare to a stallion in one breeding season.

STALL MUCKER   A person whose job is to clean stalls.

STOPPING A MARE   Getting a mare in foal.

SUTURE (*v.*)   To repair a laceration or, in mares, to partially close the vulva to prevent external contamination of the vagina, cervix and uterus.

TAIL, TAIL UP (*v.*)   Forcibly elevating the tail over an animal's back by grasping it very close to the body and pushing upward; prevents kicking in most cases.

TEAR (*n.*)   A vulvar laceration incurred during foaling or breeding.

TEASE (*v.*)   To see if a mare is in season by exposing her to a teaser.

TEASER   A male horse used to see if mares are in season.

TEN ACROSS   Ten dollars bet to win, place and show on the same horse in a race.

THIRD EYELID   The nictitating membrane, a membrane in the inner corner of horses' eyes.

THOROUGHBRED-CROSS   A horse with one Thoroughbred parent and one non-Thoroughbred parent.

TIED TONGUE OR TONGUE TIE   A strap that holds a horse's tongue in place so it won't be swallowed or interfere with the passage of air.

TRANSPORT MEDIUM   A mixture of nutrients that sustain bacterial life until a culture swab can be taken to a laboratory.

TWITCH (*n.*)   An ax handle or similar instrument with a loop of soft, thin rope on one end that is placed over a horse's upper lip and twisted, to aid in controlling the animal; (*v.*) to use a twitch.

WEANLING   In horsebreeding, a young horse from the time it is taken off its dam through December 31 of the year of birth.

WELSH PONY   A medium-size pony, roughly halfway between a Shetland Pony and a full-size horse.

WITHERS   The highest part of a horse's back, just behind the neck.

WORM, DEWORM (*v.*)   To give a medication that kills internal parasites; (*n.*) the parasite itself.

YEARLING   A one-year-old horse. Any horse between January 1 and December 31 of the year *after* it is born.